NATURAL
SLEEP

NATURAL
SLEEP

(HOW TO GET YOUR SHARE)

by Philip Goldberg and Daniel Kaufman

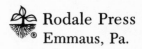 Rodale Press
Emmaus, Pa.

Printed in the United States of America on recycled paper, containing a high percentage of de-inked fiber.

Library of Congress Cataloging in Publication Data
Goldberg, Philip.
  Natural sleep.

  Bibliography: p.
  Includes index.
  1. Insomnia. I. Kaufman, Daniel, joint author.
II. Title.
RC548.G64   616.8′49   78-1745
ISBN 0-87857-216-3

2   4   6   8   10   9   7   5   3   1

ACKNOWLEDGEMENTS

We would like to express our gratitude to the many professionals who shared their knowledge with us, and were so generous with their time: Mr. Samuel Bursuk, Dr. Allan Cott, Mr. Norman Dine, Dr. Peter Hauri, Dr. Ernest Hartmann, Dr. Charles Pollack, Dr. Quentin Regestein, Dr. Elliot Weitzman. We are particularly grateful to Dr. David Viscott, whose personal encouragement and professional criticism were invaluable. Special thanks to the staff at Montefiore Hospital's Sleep-Wake Disorders Unit, who were so very cooperative, and to Mr. Covino of the Reference Staff of the Great Neck Library, New York.

We deeply appreciate the advice, support and patience that we received from our families and friends, particularly our parents, one of whom, Mrs. Ruth Lyons Kaufman, was one of the inspirations for the book, and to Jane Brodie, Jane Goldstein, Bob and Yvonne Forman, Alfred and Martha Jenkins, Mitchell Kapor, and James McVey.

We are specially indebted to the many insomniacs who shared their experiences with us; may this book put them all safely to sleep.

TO JANE

CONTENTS

What constitutes insomnia; the prevalence
of sleep disorders; shortcomings of present
literature; why this book was written; how
to use this book; comprehensive questionnaires and charts that will help the reader
to evaluate his or her own sleep and any
general health problems.

Why we sleep; what happens when we
sleep; effects of sleep loss; what causes insomnia; general considerations.

Widespread sleeping pill use; effects of
drugs on sleep and health; breaking the
sleeping pill habit; if you must use drugs.

How to deal with medical problems that
affect your sleep; physical abnormalities
requiring a doctor's attention; alcohol,
tobacco and other sleep-damaging substances; alternative physiological treatments.

for insomniacs; music and sleep; darkness; your bed and mattress; the right pillow; blankets and sheets; bedroom temperature and ventilation; Yoga and other exercises; the slant board technique; eye exercises; baths before bed.

F. Scott Fitzgerald and the legions of insomniacs; massage in bed; breathing techniques to fall asleep; hypnosis for insomniacs; relaxation techniques; the tongue-in-cheek method; roll up your eyes to bring sleep; what to do about leg jitters; put your head in the right direction; the best posture to sleep in; use your imagination in bed; what to do about snoring; miscellaneous tidbits for the sleepless.

The latest developments in sleep clinics and laboratories; interviews with leading specialists—Dr. Charles Pollack, Dr. Elliot Weitzman, Dr. Quentin Regestein, Dr. Ernest Hartmann, Dr. Peter Hauri; a patient's-eye view of a visit to a sleep center; concluding remarks.

Authors' Preface

The main purpose of this book is to help people sleep. It is, as a result, broad in range and comprehensive. We include all sensible procedures—orthodox and unorthodox—that do not involve sleeping pills, to give insomniacs the widest possible choice of pathways for finding natural sleep.

We wanted to include only those treatments that were natural. But what does that mean? The question came up early in our research. The definition that most appealed to us was, "in accordance with what is found or expected in nature." Ultimately, of course, we had to rely on our intuitive sense of what fits with nature's ways.

In some cases we were personally doubtful about the efficacy of a particular treatment. We included it anyway if it was a treatment experts take seriously. We made every effort to present the pros and cons objectively. Safety first—that was our overriding concern.

None of the instructions or suggestions in this book should be construed as a prescription for insomnia. Neither Mr. Kaufman, who conceived this project and did most of the research, nor Mr. Goldberg, who organized the material and wrote the final copy, is a medical doctor. We approached our work as journalists, attempting to be as objective as possible. We used interviews, library research, observations, and scientific evidence, as well as old wives' tales, folk remedies, serendipitous discoveries, hunches, common sense, and even rumors.

There is no one cure for insomnia. We leave it to the reader to determine for himself which of the natural procedures may be of use to him. The self-evaluating questionnaires and charts, along with the basic descriptions of the causes and effects of insomnia, will help him make intelligent choices. Any serious problems, and any questions of a medical nature, should be taken to a physician.

In addition to the practical treatments that are described, we have provided a thorough explanation of sleep, insomnia, and related topics. Though brief, those sections are up to date, and reflect the current state of scientific knowledge.

New York
October 1977

Introduction

This is a well written and amazingly complete "do-it-yourself" guide to the treatment of insomnia. I think that basically it does an excellent job.

As a scientist and a physician involved with the field of sleep, I approached the request to write an introduction with some hesitancy. As a scientist I was afraid that a book written by reporters for the general public might be so full of inaccuracies, or shortcuts to avoid difficult terminology, as to make it inaccurate and misleading. However, this does not turn out to be the case. The scientific inaccuracies here are small and are not of great importance. They do not interfere with the general meaning or flow of the book.

As a physician, of course, my concern was that such a book might lead people to try dangerous treatments, or might lead them to avoid proven medical treatments for specific medical conditions. Again, I feel that the authors have basically done a good job. They are aware that insomnia has many causes, and that some of these causes involve treatable medical and psychiatric illness, and the authors are careful to suggest in many places that consultation with a physician or with a sleep clinic may be required. There is perhaps one place where I would add a caution in addition to those provided by the authors: a sudden and drastic change in diet can sometimes be dangerous, especially in a person who has liver disease, kidney disease, or is taking various medications. The authors rightly warn of the dangers of taking drugs such as sleeping pills which can disrupt the delicate machinery of the body in many ways; unfortunately such disruption can sometimes also be caused by the sudden addition or withdrawal of natural food substances as well as by the addition of substances labeled as medications.

In its listing and discussion of "do-it-yourself" treatments for insomnia, this book is breathtakingly complete. It discusses the use of foods, diets, bedtime rituals, exercise, massage, breathing techniques, relaxation, hypnosis, herbal remedies, regularity of habits, and even such things as types of sheets, blankets and bedrooms. All this makes fascinating reading, for the good sleeper as well as the insomniac, and I learned a number of things I had not known before. I am slightly disturbed by the shotgun approach in which hundreds of possible remedies are suggested to the reader, with fairly well-established and scientifically based treatments handled in more or less the same way as really "far out" and unlikely forms of help. However, I must admit that even the most "far out" and illogical-sounding approach has probably sometimes helped someone to sleep, and I suppose we must trust the good sense of the reader to pick and choose what appears probable to him or her from the amazing wealth of possibilities presented.

I agree strongly with the authors' stand that most sleeping pills are dangerous substances and have been overused. My own position is that clearly insomnia is not an illness for which a sleeping pill is a cure (though it has too frequently been misinterpreted in this sense). Insomnia is a symptom of many underlying conditions, and the insomniac or his physician should attempt to determine the underlying cause of the insomnia and to treat that cause. Most often the cause will be behavioral-psychological, psychiatric (anxiety or depression) or medical, and the treatment will either involve no medication, or will involve medication aimed at a specific medical or psychiatric condition, rather than a sleeping pill. There is a place for the use of sleeping pills but it is a fairly limited place; even for this limited role, I believe we have not developed drugs in the right way. Sleeping pills so far have been nonspecific central nervous system depressants which have little to do with the physiology of sleep. I have recently done a great deal of research work, mentioned by the authors of this book, on a more "natural" substance which is not a nervous system depressant but is related to the physiology of sleep. This is a natural food substance, the amino acid l-tryptophan. I discuss my views of sleep, insomnia, and sleeping pills in my book *The Sleeping Pill* (Yale University Press, New Haven, 1978).

Overall, I believe this book, *Natural Sleep*, may be of help to a number of persons suffering from mild or moderate insomnia who will find in it something directly useful to them. In addition, the book is fun to read.

Ernest Hartmann, M.D.
Director, Sleep and Dream Laboratory
Boston State Hospital

Professor of Psychiatry
Tufts University School of Medicine

Medical Director,
Sleep Research Foundation

A flock of sheep that leisurely pass by,
One after one; the sound of rain, and bees
murmuring; the fall of rivers, winds
    and seas,
Smooth fields, white sheets of water,
    and pure sky,
I have thought of all by turns and yet
    do lie
Sleepless! . . .
Come, blessed barrier between day
    and day
Dear mother of fresh thoughts
    and joyous health!

—William Wordsworth

How many thousand of my poorest subjects
Are at this hour asleep!
    O sleep, O gentle sleep,
Nature's soft nurse, how have I frighted thee,
That thou no more wilt weigh my eyelids down
And steep my senses in forgetfulness?

Shakespeare (*Henry IV, Part II*)

CHAPTER ONE

EVALUATING YOUR SLEEP PROBLEM

Nature evolves in regular, pulsating rhythms. From the tiniest atoms to huge clusters of galaxies, each unit of creation vibrates in cyclical fashion—up-down, in-out, stop-go. Within our bodies are over one hundred different cycles whose regular patterns affect the metabolism of our cells, the pumping of our blood, the intake of oxygen, and even our moods and our states of consciousness. When these cycles mesh appropriately with one another and with the rhythms of their environments our well being and progress are assured, for then we are functioning as nature intended. When the rhythms are out of synchrony, then, as in an orchestra, cacophony results. The body suffers.

The periodicity of these syncopated biological rhythms ranges from a fraction of a second to a number of years. Some, like the sleep/wake cycle that is the concern of this book, are called *circadian*, from the Latin circa (approximately) and diés (days). These cycles obey the daily pattern set down by the rotation of the earth, taking approximately 24 hours to run their course.

Evening falls and flowers fold their petals. Plants fold their leaves. With the exception of owls and other nighttime predators, the creatures of land, sea, and air all curl up into

1

bedroom niches in the rocks and trees and sand. Dawn comes and the unfolding begins. The outside world, which had been barred from the senses of the sleepers, is once again admitted.

It is the most natural thing in the world, intended no doubt to be accomplished effortlessly. Yet, a growing number of people find themselves alarmingly disconnected from the natural flow of sleeping and waking that nature intended us to follow.

How many people suffer from insomnia? The estimates vary, ranging from 20 million to 50 million Americans—from 10 to 25 percent of the population. That's a lot of tossing and turning, even if we accept the most conservative estimate. And those estimates usually are based on the number of *serious* insomniacs, the definition of which varies considerably. Some doctors define insomniacs as those who can't sleep *at all;* others are willing to categorize as insomniacs all those who complain about their sleep. The currently accepted definition, sure to become known as DIMS, is: "Difficulty initiating or maintaining sleep."

Several surveys have tried to pin down the exact incidence of sleep problems. Of 1,000 households surveyed in Los Angeles, one third had someone with current problems, and in 42 percent someone suffered with sleep problems at some time. *Esquire* magazine describes a Gallup poll in which 50 percent of those interviewed had trouble falling asleep or staying asleep. In Gainesville, Florida, psychiatrist Ismet Karacan surveyed 1,645 people and found that a third to one-half had trouble sleeping. A University of California survey indicates that one-third of the population has recurrent bouts with insomnia, and 15 percent suffer with it chronically.

Polls of doctors have also been revealing, though somewhat disparate. In one survey, roughly 19 percent of the patients seen by the 3,000 doctors queried had complaints of insomnia (Figure 1). That figure may be understating the case, for some say that more people in the United States visit doctors for help getting to sleep than for any other single complaint. It is also said that half of those not considered insomniacs have a sleepless night on occasion, and a large, but undetermined number do not sleep as efficiently as they should.

DOCTORS ESTIMATE INSOMNIA INCIDENCE AMONG PATIENTS

Type of practice	Incidence of insomnia
Family practice	12.8 percent
Gastroenterology and cardiovascular disease	18.3 percent
General practice	14.0 percent
Internal medicine	17.5 percent
Neurology	14.1 percent
Obstetrics and gynecology	11.6 percent
Pediatrics	15.5 percent
Psychiatry	33.2 percent
Surgery	16.4 percent
Child psychiatry	18.6 percent
Average	18.7 percent

Figure 1. Responses from 3,000 physicians to survey by Dr. Anthony Kales.

Insomniacs can take comfort in knowing that they are in excellent company, even if it does feel lonely in that dark room. As you toss and turn, count sheep, make lists, or play word games; as you try to still your mind; as you contemplate what a lousy day tomorrow will be if you don't fall asleep immediately; as you inch dangerously closer to the medicine chest you might be accompanied by as many as 50 million of your countrymen. That's a veritable epidemic.

You are also part of a venerable tradition. While we have no way of knowing how prevalent the affliction has been in the past, the legends and lore of nearly every known culture bewail the torment of those unable to sleep. The evidence suggests that magical potions, herbs, esoteric rituals, and incantations specifically designed to induce sleep in the sleepless have been used for thousands of years. The tombs of ancient Pharaohs, wherein all things considered indispensable for the living were lodged, are said to have contained urns of sleep-promoting herbs, such as chamomile, lest the spirit of the departed monarch suffer a sleepless night. Ancient Egyptian hieroglyphs record a lament for three living hells, one of which is, "to be in bed and sleep not."

From our own cultural heritage, the present day insomniac can claim as restless bedfellow the Roman poet Horace, who coined the phrase "I cannot sleep a wink," over 2,000 years ago. Proust, Kafka, Kipling, Nietzsche, and Poe are but a few of the notables whose writings record bouts with insomnia. So was the irrepressible Mark Twain, who has supplied us with enough quips on the subject to enable us to laugh our way to sleep. So many of Shakespeare's characters lyrically toss and turn across the pages of his plays that one twentieth century pedant was moved to write a book titled, *Shakespeare's Insomnia*. The list of sleepless wonders includes dozens of noteworthy artists, statesmen, scientists, and others whose contributions might not have been made had they slept as much as most of us think we should.

Those starved by what Shakespeare called the "chief nourisher of life's feast" come in three basic categories: the most prevalent are those who cannot fall asleep upon going to bed and who remain awake for what usually seems an eternity, even though they feel exhausted mentally and physically. This type of insomnia is termed *initial* insomnia by clinicians.

The second type was well described by Franz Kafka: "I fall asleep soundly, but after an hour I wake up, as though I had laid my head in the wrong hole. I ... have before me anew the labour of falling asleep and feel myself rejected by sleep." Called *intermittent* insomnia, this type may recur any number of times in a given night, and seems to be more prevalent among the middle-aged and elderly, especially those with physical disorders.

In the third category—*matutinal* or *terminal* insomnia—are those who fall asleep well enough but wake up prematurely, usually after five or six hours, dull, weary, unrefreshed, and unable to fall back to sleep.

Some authorities add a category for those who simply do not sleep well. That is, they fall asleep fairly promptly, awaken after a reasonable length of time, say, seven or eight hours, but are not as refreshed as they should be, and are fatigued during the day. Their sleep is inefficient. That category may include many of us (perhaps a large majority) who would never think of calling ourselves insomniacs.

There is reasonable evidence to suggest that we are, as a

nation, chronically deprived of proper sleep.

With the advent of electric lights, human beings began to break from the rest of nature, engaging in stimulating activity later and later into the night. Television and other entertainment opportunities further aggravated the pattern. Yet, unlike our ancestors who typically went to sleep not long after sundown, we tend to get up when we must, not when we want to or feel a natural need to. In an article in the *Bulletin of Psychosomatic Society*, Drs. W. B. Webb and H. W. Agnew reported several studies to support the notion that we are chronically sleep deprived: the sleep of young students surveyed in 1910 and 1911 was 1½ hours longer than a 1963 comparison group; a recent survey of 1,000 students revealed that a third "find it very hard to get up in the morning," and less than a third woke up refreshed and rested. Other surveys revealed that students typically sleep an hour longer on weekends, and that when left on their own in a schedule-free situation, they exceeded their usual sleep by more than an hour.

If you have picked up this book for any reason other than idle curiosity, the chances are you frequently or occasionally have difficulty sleeping. Or, you may be a reasonably good sleeper who is interested in improving the quality of your sleep or in avoiding the occasional sleepless night that each of us encounters due to unusual situations—travel, an important event, illness, excessive pressure at work, or a tragedy. In every case we are sure you will benefit from the practical suggestions in this book.

Why the Book Was Written

Both authors were chronic insomniacs at one time. Like our fellow sleepless wonders—perhaps like you—we reached for the handiest remedy—sleeping pills—when first confronted with the problem. We used both prescribed and over-the-counter varieties and soon suffered the mental and physical ravages typical among users and abusers of sleep medication, ravages which are described fully later on. Subsequently, our sleep unimproved, we sought natural ways of dealing with sleeplessness and its consequences.

When we first began to seek out alternatives to drugs we discovered that there was a striking need for a comprehensive compendium of natural ways to improve sleep. There was plenty of literature on sleep and insomnia, all of which counselled against the use of drugs, but they were mainly technical in nature—usually scholarly tomes explaining the current state of theoretical and scientific knowledge on the subjects.

Some books offered practical suggestions for combatting insomnia. These, however, were either out of date, or heavily weighted toward one, or perhaps a few, of the numerous approaches to sleep problems.

Others were devoted exclusively to hackneyed, often banal platitudes that can be summarized by "learn to relax" or "don't worry." Good advice, but hardly practical, concrete, or comprehensive, and certainly not enough to coax a restless nervous system into the arms of "Nature's soft nurse," as Shakespeare called sleep.

We ended up consulting a wide variety of sources and experimenting with a wide variety of treatments. Our research helped with our own sleep problems considerably. We still have our difficult nights, but they come with far less frequency and severity. We are no longer *chronic* insomniacs. Rather, we have joined the enviable members of the population who have to do battle with an elusive sandman only on occasion.

When we decided to write this book, we added to our own experiences all the material we could gather from copious reading and interviewing. The result is a how-to oriented handbook that should aid everyone from the severe insomniac to the average person who wants to make the most of those mysterious nighttime hours.

In our investigations we learned that science has only recently gotten around to the serious study of sleep and sleep disorders. Sleep research is off to an auspicious start. But, like all new areas of inquiry, this one is filled with contradictory opinions, promising theories, wild speculation, and even controversy. It is moving along at the same agonizingly slow pace with which sleep seems to come to insomniacs. The methods of science require complex, time-consuming processes of experimentation and repeated validation.

But time is not the only hindrance to science's understanding of insomnia. We found that physicians—for reasons we cannot comprehend—are, as a whole, resistant to the simple notion of looking to nature for guidance. Perhaps because this is an age of technology, we seem to gravitate toward the complex and cumbersome rather than to follow the simple and economical, as nature does. Thus, sleep research has largely ignored such obvious areas of importance as nutrition, choosing instead to experiment with elaborate technology and abstract psychological contrivances.

Science's approach to sleep problems has been hampered by the same narrow perspective that has dominated our approach to health in general, and that has made us a nation of promiscuous pill-poppers. We view parts in isolation, without regard to the whole. Thus, for all its magnificent achievements, medical science has structured its healing arts almost entirely on the treatment of specific, discrete symptoms.

Headaches, to use a typical example, are treated with pills to cover up the pain. Little attention is given, at least by the average doctor, to the emotions, behavior, diet, or general physical health, all factors that might result in headaches. Only recently have we considered treating the whole person. We have paid scant attention to fundamental, underlying causes—or to the complex interdependence of different areas of the body, or, especially, to the prevention of ailments. Thus, insomnia has been treated, for the most part, with sleeping pills.

Now that the deleterious effects of sleep drugs have become evident, the medical community is looking for alternatives. So far, not much has been uncovered, although the field looks more promising all the time. Clearly, however, those reasonable alternatives that exist have not been adequately researched or reported. It is significant that scientists who had been trying to isolate one magical cure-all for insomnia, are fast learning that a broader, more holistic view of the problem—and of health in general—is imperative.

In ancient, traditional cultures the healing arts tended to view symptoms as indications of a more general malfunction involving the body as a whole. In this view all parts of the organism affect all other parts. Mind, behavior, environment, and body all fit together in an organic, interconnected way to make up a unified whole that is more than a collection of parts. Nothing can be ignored when treating any ailment.

This is especially true, we are discovering, with something as fundamental as sleep. A headache, a virus, a broken toe, or an infection should, of course, be treated holistically. But, in those cases, the immediate treatment of the symptom, and its efficacious removal, makes more sense than it does with insomnia. Insomnia is not a disease; it is a *sign*, or, as sleep specialists like to say, it is a *complaint*. Always, it is symptomatic of other factors, sometimes superficial and mundane; sometimes deep and serious.

One person's sleep problems may be caused by factors entirely different from those keeping the next person awake, even though the symptoms may appear to be identical. Most experts agree that sleep difficulties are usually multi-faceted. What happens when your head hits the pillow at night depends, in some way, on everything you did, said, felt, thought, ate, drank, and experienced from the moment you raised your head off the pillow that morning. Indeed, it is affected by every prior moment of your life. For those reasons, diagnosis is always an individual matter.

In the process of doing our research we tried to keep those points in mind. And we tried to maintain a holistic perspective. We urge the reader to do the same. When we turned to experts we discovered, to our delight, that there is a growing number of individuals—physicians, psychologists, nutritionists and others—whose perspectives are widening, and whose minds are open to alternatives to traditional medicine. They are uncovering much that is useful and natural with which to supplement their orthodox methods. It was from those persons that we received much of our information. We balanced that information with standard medical opinion.

Our status as fellow-sufferers, we felt, had several advantages. It enabled us personally to try out some of the methods discussed, and it provided us with a good deal of empathy. One of the problems with insomnia is that it elicits very little sympathy from others, even from friends.

"I hardly slept a wink," does not elicit the same response as "I have the flu," or even, "I stubbed my toe." No one writes doleful tunes about the sleepless, and no one will ever make a tear-jerking movie about a nonsleeper. Insomnia is rarely an acceptable excuse for being absent, late, forgetful, or lazy. There are no outward signs with which to elicit sympathy: no sneezes, no blood, no plaster casts to autograph, no scars to show off, no impressive Latin terms to drop. More often than not insomniacs encounter not sympathy, but antipathy—even from their own spouses who are likely to complain about all the tossing and turning.

Most afflictions are thought of as unavoidable impositions from the outside. "Poor thing," the sufferer is told, "It could have happened to anyone." Not so with insomnia. Like an unhappy marriage or body odor, it is usually considered self-inflicted and avoidable. Insomniacs can't file for disability if their sleep loss ends up getting them fired. Nor is insomnia enough of an excuse for being bad company. And no one sends insomniacs get well cards.

Having spent a good deal of time imprisoned by insomnia we know what it's like to go through a day with bleary eyes and rubbery knees. And we know what helped us. Therefore, the book emphasizes practical suggestions. We are convinced that insomnia can be licked naturally, and with relative ease.

In most cases, you can do it yourself.

"The insomniac patient should be made to understand that he or she must take charge of his own life," states sleep expert, Dr. Quentin Regestein. "Don't take your body to the doctor as if he were a repair shop."

How to Use This Book

The first three chapters will give you a basic understanding of the function of sleep, the causes of insomnia, and the effects of drugs. This will provide a foundation for properly evaluating and applying the methods available for aiding sleep. Those methods, along with the guidance of your physician or psychologist when necessary, plus your own awareness of your particular needs and problems, will bring welcome relief. More than likely it will bring complete recovery, from even chronic sleeplessness. At the very least, it will point you in the direction of the kind of assistance you need.

The treatments and suggestions that begin in chapter four are divided into categories for convenience. In some cases, the category assignment is somewhat arbitrary. A practice recommended for bedtime, for example, might also be employed during the day or when you are awakened during sleep. In such instances, the procedure appears in the category in which it is most likely to be used, and other suggested applications are mentioned.

We want to suggest several things to do while reading the book to make the most of the information. We recommend that you underline, take notes, or in some other way annotate as you go along. Nothing formal. Just follow your instincts, noting the points that strike a familiar chord or stand out in any way, however vague. Chances are you will note points that will be of greatest value to you.

Perhaps you will find that you identify with certain symptoms of insomnia. Or perhaps one of the factors that causes insomnia sort of jumps at you from the page. Maybe some recognition will come when you are reading about some of the methods of treatment—perhaps a vitamin or a bedtime ritual strikes you as particularly fascinating. Note that. It might be engaging your attention because it has practical value for you. Trust your intuition. Ultimately, you are the only one who can determine which of the many methods you should try. Looking back over your notes and underlinings will give you good clues.

Since every person's sleep needs are different, it is important to understand yourself and your own sleep patterns thoroughly. Most of us think we know ourselves as well as we need to, but, often, a little help in getting a closer look at our inner selves goes a long way. For that reason we have included charts and questionnaires for you to fill out while reading this book. You will be surprised at how much more aware you will be of your sleep problems, and the factors that may be affecting them, just because you took time out to consider your responses.

Some of the questionnaires can be filled out as soon as you come to them. We recommend doing so before you go on with the next chapter. Others are meant to serve as running logs. These should be kept daily and continued for at least two weeks. The greater personal awareness the charts will elicit should make your notations later in the book all the more valid.

When you have finished the book, go back over all your charts and questionnaires. Then skim the book, paying particular attention to the sections you singled out. Then you will be in a good position to judge which combination of methods will best fit your needs. Your case might call for nothing more than an eyeshade or a little more exercise. Or you might need a radical change in diet or other habits. You might even need to visit a sleep clinic. In any case, if you pay attention to your responses to the questionnaires, and if you read carefully, you are bound to end up sleeping more soundly and spending less time and money on doing so.

For example, you may notice in your sleep log that you awaken at the same time every night, unable to fall back to sleep. If so, your reading may show you that your main problem was believing you had a problem, and that a simple change of schedule might help.

On the other hand, you may have noted that your spouse complains of being kicked during the night. When you read about myoclonic seizures in chapter five, perhaps you put two and two together and concluded that only a sleep clinic can help.

To solve most cases some experimentation is required. Pick and choose. Make educated guesses. Discuss your ideas with your family, friends and trusted health experts. Consider your budget. And be objective. Don't try so many things at the same time that you can't tell what's doing what. On the other hand, if you have a problem that is of major concern, don't fiddle around too long and don't spare the expense. Sleep is one of your best friends. Treat it generously.

PERSONAL SLEEP QUESTIONNAIRE

This questionnaire will make you more aware of your sleep patterns, your habits, and your problems. Reference will be made to each point throughout the book.

1. Do you sleep soundly?
   Usually _____   Sometimes _____   Never _____

2. Do you awaken in the night?
   Usually _____   Sometimes _____   Never _____

   If so, how many times per night? _____
   For how long? _____
   _____

3. Do you ever awaken too early in the morning unable to return to sleep?
   Usually _____   Sometimes _____   Never _____

4. How much sleep do you get on the average night?
   _____
   Has that changed? _____
   If so, when? _____
   _____

5. What is your usual bedtime?
   Before 10 P.M.   Between 10 and 12
   Between 12 and 2 A.M.   After 2 A.M.

   5a. Are you usually tired at bedtime? _____
   5b. Do you stay up long after you are sleepy? _____
   _____
   _____

6. What time do you usually wake up?
   Before 6 A.M.   Between 8 and 10
   Between 6 and 8   After 10 A.M.

7. Do you usually go to bed at the same time each night?
   _____
   _____

8. Do you usually get up at the same time each morning?
   _____
   _____

9. Have either your bedtime or your waking times changed recently? _____
   When? _____
   Explain the change _____
   _____
   _____

10. How do you usually feel when you get out of bed in the morning?
    _____ Alert, wide awake
    _____ Awake, but not fully alert
    _____ Foggy
    _____ Still sleepy. Want to sleep more.
    10a. Has this changed? _____
    When? _____
    Explain the change: _____
    _____
    _____
    How do you account for it? _____
    _____
    10b. Do you use an alarm clock? _____
    _____

11. How long does it take you to fall asleep once you get into bed?
    _____ less than 15 minutes
    _____ 15-30 minutes
    _____ 30-45 minutes
    _____ 45 minutes to an hour
    _____ More than an hour
    11a. Has this changed? _____
    When? _____
    Explain the change _____
    _____
    _____
    How do you account for it? _____
    _____
    11b. What do you think about when lying awake?
    _____
    11c. What do you feel physically? _____
    _____

12. Do you feel that you get enough sleep? _____

(continued next page)

13. When did you last fall asleep easily? _____

14. When did you last sleep well through the night?

_____

15. When did you last wake up refreshed? _____

16. If your sleep pattern has changed, what do you think
    caused it? _____

_____

17. How do you account for your sleep problems? _____

_____

18. Do you take sleeping pills?
    ____ Prescription?   ____ Over-the-counter?
    18a. How often do you take them? _____
    18b. How long have you been taking them? _____

19. What other medication do you take? _____

20. Do you drink alcohol? _____
    How much per day? _____

21. Do you smoke cigarettes? _____
    How many per day? _____

22. Do you drink coffee? _____
    How many cups per day? _____

23. Do you have any medical problems?

_____

    What are they? _____

_____

24. What do you do when you are unable to sleep at night?

_____

25. During the day, do you ever worry about whether you
    will sleep that night? _____

_____

26. Do you take naps during the day? _____
    How often? _____ For how long? _____
    At what time of day? _____
    26a. Do you often feel like napping but do not have
         the opportunity? _____
    At what time of day? _____
    26b. Has this changed? _____
    When? _____
    Why? _____

27. Do you think that most people sleep better than you do?

_____

28. How many hours of sleep does the average person get?
_____

29. How much sleep do human beings need? _____
_____

30. What do you think is the most common cause of insomnia? _____

31. Do you snore?
Usually ____   Sometimes ____   Never ____
Softly ____   Loudly ____

32. Does your spouse complain of being kicked in the night?
Usually ____   Sometimes ____   Never ____

33. Do you have trouble breathing during your sleep?
_____

34. Is your bedroom noisy? _____
State the noise problem. _____
_____

What do you do about the noise problem? _____
_____
_____

35. Is your bedroom dark? _____
Are you bothered by light in the morning? _____

36. Is the air in your bedroom too humid?   Too dry?
Too warm?   Too cold?

37. Do you sleep alone? _____
If not, do you use twin beds or a double bed?

38. Are your covers too heavy?   Too short?
Too binding?

39. Are you too cold at night?   Too warm?

40. Is your mattress comfortable?   Too soft?
Too hard?

41. What posture do you sleep in? _____

42. Do you bring work home with you on a regular basis?
_____

43. How do you usually spend your last hour before going to bed? _____

44. Do you do anything to help you fall asleep?
Bath?   Relaxation technique?
Foods or drinks?   Exercises?   Music?
Other _____

STRESS FACTORS

The following is a list of life changes known to produce stress. It was compiled in 1965 by Dr. T. H. Holmes, a psychiatrist from the University of Washington, and it goes from the most stressful changes to the least stressful. Which of these events has occurred in your life? For each "yes" write

Event	yes or no	date occurred	sleep change? yes no	how?
Death of Spouse				
Divorce				
Marital Separation				
Jail Term				
Death of close family member				
Personal injury or illness				
Getting married				
Fired at Work				
Reconciliation with mate				
Retirement				
Changed health in family member				
Pregnancy				
Sex difficulties				
Gaining a new family member				
Business readjustment				
Change in financial status				
Death of a close friend				
Change to a different line of work				
Increase in arguments with mate				
Mortgage over $10,000.00*				
Foreclosure of mortgage or loan				
Change in work responsibility				

*Figure reflects housing costs of 1965. Adjust for inflation rate in your area.

how long ago it occurred, and whether you noticed any change in your sleep immediately thereafter.

These stress factors often lead to disturbed sleep. Recalling which of these changes you have been exposed to may help you identify the cause of situational insomnia. Often, insomnia is precipitated by a real event, and is then perpetuated for reasons discussed later on.

Event	yes or no	date occurred	sleep change? yes no	how?
Child leaving home				
Trouble with in-laws				
Outstanding personal achievement				
Mate begins or ends work				
Change in living conditions				
Revision of personal habits				
Trouble with boss				
Changed work hours or conditions				
Change in residence				
Change in schools				
Change in recreation				
Change in church activities				
Change in social activities				
Mortgage or loan under $10,000.00*				
Changed number of family meetings				
Change in sleeping habits				
Change in eating habits				
Vacation				
Christmas				
Minor violation of law				

DIET CHART

In chapter 6, we discuss the nutritional causes of insomnia, and the ways in which dietary treatments can help improve sleep. To make the most of that information, we suggest that you keep the following log—it will help you become more aware of your diet, and thus to make useful changes.

Every day for the next two weeks, or until you finish reading this book, keep track of *everything* you eat and drink.

DAY 1   **Breakfast** (note time)
Food   Drink

Snacks (note time)
Food   Drink

Lunch (note time)
Food   Drink

Snacks (note time)
Food   Drink

Supper (note time)
Food   Drink

Snacks (note time)
Food   Drink

What time did you go to bed?
At bedtime, did you feel bloated?   full?   comfortable?
   slightly hungry?   starving?   stomach upset?

Place a * next to anything that contains caffeine (coffee, tea, cola, chocolate).

Place a + next to anything that contains sugar.

Place a X next to all starchy food (breads, potatoes, macaroni, etc.).

Place a 0 next to foods you salted.

GENERAL HEALTH

Medical factors contribute to sleep problems. These questions will help you identify possible problems with your health and diet. This is, of course, not meant to substitute in any way for a doctor's examination. It is just to help raise your awareness of your health.

1. Have you been to a doctor recently?

   For any particular complaint?

   What?

2. List all serious illnesses in your life.

3. List any recent ailments, even minor.

4. Do you consider yourself a healthy person?

5. Do you exercise regularly?

GENERAL HEALTH QUESTIONNAIRE

Instructions: Use figures (1) *Mild;* (2) *Moderate;* (3) *Severe* to show degrees of severity. IF ANY PART of question applies, indicate as above.

1. ( ) Stool shows undigested foods?

2. ( ) Long history of constipation?

3. ( ) Indigestion (fullness, bloating, sourness) occurs two or three hours after meals?

4. ( ) Indigestion occurs immediately after eating?

5. ( ) Heavy, full logy feeling after eating heavy meat meal?

6. ( ) Excessive lower bowel gas (flatulence)?

7. ( ) Stomach *pain* occurs five or six hours after eating, usually at night, relieved by eating or drinking milk or cream?

8. ( ) Diarrhea occurs frequently?

9. ( ) Blood pressure fluctuates, has been "too high" on occasion?

10. ( ) Have you had frequent or severe attacks of pneumonia, bronchitis, flu, sinusitis?

11. ( ) Have you had allergies, such as skin rash, dermatitis, hay fever, severe sneezing attacks, asthma or other allergy?

12. ( ) Do you have an unusual craving for salt?

13. ( ) Do you have an unusual craving for sugar?

14. ( ) Do you perspire excessively?

15. ( ) Have you had persistent high blood pressure to the best of your knowledge?

16. ( ) People remark that you "breathe loudly," are heard breathing in quiet room?

17. ( ) Feel dizzy or nauseated in morning?

18. ( ) Gain weight, fail to lose weight on diets?

19. ( ) Difficulty concentrating, easily distracted?

20. ( ) Do you have a strong drive followed by exhaustion, repeated in cycles?

21. ( ) Does protruding tongue quiver, hands shake?

22. ( ) Night sweats, wake up frightened?

23. ( ) Muscle weakness, weak grip, weak legs, objects feel unusually heavy?

24. ( ) Feel drowsy, chronic fatigue?

25. ( ) Cold hands and feet, use extra clothing, bed-clothing, heat pads to keep warm?

26. ( ) Nervousness, shaky feeling, headaches are relieved by eating sweets?

27. ( ) Irritable if late for a meal, if meal is missed, before breakfast?

28. ( ) Experience sudden strong craving for sweets, alcohol?

29. ( ) Get hungry "five minutes after eating?"

30. ( ) Wake up at night feeling hungry often?

31. ( ) Chronic fatigue, lowered resistence?

32. ( ) Ever shown sugar in urine, or been diagnosed as a diabetic?

PERSONAL SLEEP RECORD

Throughout the book we discuss many points that are relevant to people with particular sleep patterns and idiosyn-
crasies. This log will make you more conscious of your own.

Starting tonight, fill in this chart every day for the next
week or until you finish the book, whichever is longer.

Instructions:

Mark the time you went to bed with an arrow pointing
down (↓).

Mark the time you think you fell asleep with a red dot.

Mark the times you woke up (during the night or in the
morning) with a green dot.

Mark the times you got out of bed with an arrow pointing
up (↑).

Mark daytime naps in the same manner or with an N.

Day	Date	10 PM	11 PM	Midn't	1 AM	2 AM	etc.

	Day
Each day answer the following questions:	

1. How long did it take you to fall asleep?

2. How many times did you wake up?

3. How much total sleep time did you get?

4. Did you *have* to be up at a certain time? What time?

5. Did you use an alarm?

6. On a scale of a) very tired b) somewhat tired c) OK d) alert e) very alert

   How did you feel first thing in the morning?

   How did you feel two hours after waking?

   How did you feel at lunchtime?

   How did you feel two hours after lunch?

   How did you feel at dinner time?

   How did you feel two hours after dinner?

   How did you feel at bedtime?

PSYCHOLOGICAL FACTORS

In chapter seven, and elsewhere in the book, we discuss the attitudes and emotional problems that contribute to insomnia. These questions will help you evaluate those factors in your own life.

1. Do you tend to worry a lot? _____
   What things worry you?
      —your health?
      —loss of love?
      —loss of money?
      —death?
      —others?

2. Do you get depressed? _____
   Often ____   Sometimes ____   Never ____
   What depresses you? _____
   _____

3. Do you get nervous anticipating a difficult day? _____
   _____

4. Are you thought of as ambitious? _____

5. Are you impatient? _____

6. Are you often restless? _____

7. Do you find it hard to relax? _____

8. Do you enjoy competition? _____
   Do you fear it? _____

9. Are you aggressive? _____

10. Are you unable to separate work from play? _____

11. Do you take your problems home with you? _____
    Do you take your problems to bed with you? _____

12. Do you drive yourself too hard? _____

13. Do you take time to relax? _____

14. Do you argue with your family? _____

    Do you argue at night? _____

15. Are you known as a person with a good sense of humor?

    _____

16. Do you seek the respect of others? _____

    _____

    Do you fear losing it? _____

    _____

17. Are you easily hurt? _____

    When was the last time someone hurt you? _____

    _____

    Explain what happened. _____

    _____

    _____

    _____

18. Do you get angry?
    Often ____   Sometimes ____   Seldom ____

    What angers you? _____

    _____

    Do you express your anger or do you hold it in?

    _____

19. Do you face your problems squarely? _____

    Do you tend to make excuses? _____

    _____

    Do you pretend things are going well when they are
    not? _____

    _____

20. Have you ever had psychiatric treatment? _____

    How long? _____

    _____

    Why did you go? _____

    _____

    Why did you stop? _____

    _____

(continued next page)

21. Are you easily startled or shaken up? _____
_____

    What causes that? _____

22. Do you cry easily? _____
    Do you tend to keep your sadness to yourself? ___
_____

23. Do you lose your temper easily? _____
_____

24. Do you respond well to pressure? _____
_____

    Or do you "go to pieces?" _____
_____

25. Do you have trouble letting go and enjoying
yourself? _____

CHAPTER TWO

THE BEDTIME STORY

> Now, blessings light on him that first invented
> sleep! It covers a man all over, thoughts and all,
> like a cloak; it is meat for the hungry, drink for
> the thirsty, heat for the cold and cold for the hot.
> It is the current coin that purchases all the
> pleasures of the world cheap, and the balance
> that sets the king and the shepherd, the fool and
> the wise man even.
>
> —Cervantes

Few of us can say it with the poetic grace of Cervantes,
but we are all aware that we need to sleep, just as we need
oxygen or food.

Just why this is so remains a mystery to science. Why is
sleep necessary? How much of it do we need? How do we fall
asleep? What goes on in our bodies and minds during sleep?
Why is it that some of us do not sleep well?

We know, essentially, what goes on when we breathe
and when we eat. Now we want to know the same about
sleep.

To obtain the answers to these questions, a growing
amount of time, energy and money is being devoted to
research in sleep laboratories and clinics across the country.

By monitoring the physiological processes that occur
during sleep, by studying the effects of sleep deprivation,
changes in natural sleep patterns over time, differences in
sleep habits among different groups of people under different

conditions, and by studying the sleep of animals, researchers are uncovering a great deal of information. But they still do not have a complete, precise, irrefutable set of answers.

A report from the sleep clinic at New York's Montefiore Hospital states: "Beginnings have been made in answering questions about what sleep is, what functions it serves, and of how people fall asleep, awaken, and remain awake. Despite these promising beginnings, however, virtually the whole field of sleep remains to be explored."

What Happens When We Sleep?

At one time scientists believed that in sleep all bodily functions shut down completely. Not so. It turns out that sleep is a highly dynamic state, nearly as active, nearly as complex as ordinary waking consciousness. During sleep, the bodily system as a whole follows a regular, oscillating cycle,

A NORMAL NINETY MINUTE SLEEP CYCLE	Stage	Brain Waves
	Threshold of sleep	Steady, even alpha rhythms 9–12 cycles per second.
	Stage I	Smaller, slower, pinched, irregular, variable.
	Stage II	Larger, occasional quick bursts.
	Stage III	Slow, large (5 times as big as stage I), about one per second.
	Stage IV	Very large delta waves; slow, jagged pattern.
	REM	Irregular, small, big bursts, resembles waking.

one that differs only insignificantly from one person to another. Scientists have distinguished two distinct stages of sleep, each as different from the other as either is from the waking state. These are called REM and non-REM (or NREM). The distinctions will be clear in a moment.

When you first fall asleep, you slip into NREM sleep, which then proceeds in four discrete stages (see figure 1). In Stage I, the muscles start to relax, breathing becomes regular, body temperature begins to fall, but the sleeper, on the border of wakefulness, can be aroused easily, and might even claim not to have been asleep at all. It is a shallow stage of sleep.

During Stages II and III, sleep becomes progressively deeper. The body processes slow down still further, and it becomes more and more difficult to waken the sleeper. In Stage IV, the deepest stage of sleep, breathing is even; heart rate, blood pressure, and body temperature are all low and still falling.

Behavior and experiences	Depth of sleep	Bodily activity
Relaxation, mind wanders, awareness dull.	Borderline.	Slowing down, muscular tension decreasing.
Drifting thoughts and dreams, floating feeling.	Easily awakened, might deny having slept.	Gradual slowing down, pulse growing more even, breathing more regular, temperature falling.
Some thought-like fragments; eyes will not see if opened.	Easily awakened by sounds.	Continued decrease of all bodily functions (blood pressure, metabolism, secretions, pulse, etc.), eyes may roll slowly from side to side.
More removed from outer world, rarely able to recall thoughts or dreams.	More difficult to awaken—takes louder noise.	All processes continue to drop.
Virtual oblivion, poor recall; a rare nightmare; if a sleep walker or bed wetter, those begin now.	Very difficult to awaken; the deepest sleep.	Continued decrease to deepest state of physical rest.
Rapid eye movements, dreaming vividly about 85% of the time.	Difficult to bring back to reality.	Chin muscles slack; blood pressure, pulse, breath irregular; penile erections; toes and fingers may twitch.

Then comes what is called the REM state, after the Rapid Eye Movements that occur just as though the sleeper were watching something. This is the state in which most dreaming occurs, and has, in fact, become synonymous with the dream state. The bodily processes change more radically— the sleeper is limp, the chin muscles are slack, but blood pressure, heart rate, and respiratory rate, all of which had lowered during the four NREM stages, elevate, becoming more variable. The brain-wave patterns, which had gradually become larger, smoother and slower, now begin to resemble the active, irregular patterns of the waking state.

The evidence indicates that a higher level of mental and nervous system activity goes on during REM. It had once been thought that the rapid eye movements and the penile erections that occur at that time were reactions to the contents of dreams. This has since been refuted. "It is now realized," states a publication from Montefiore's clinic, "that rapid eye movements and penile erections are caused by centers of the brain that differ from those that produce dreams. Thus the physiological behavior characteristic of REM is not caused by mental activity but goes on at the same time as the mental activity."

These cycles—beginning with NREM and ending with REM*—proceed in cycles of 90 to 100 minutes in duration. About four or five such cycles occur during the average night's sleep. Everyone, whether an insomniac or a normal sleeper, follows these basic patterns. The differences lie in the amount of time spent in the various stages; poor sleepers tend to spend less time in the valuable Stage IV and REM states, and also to have the cycles disrupted more frequently by periods of wakefulness. (With aging, the amount of total sleep, REM sleep, and Stage III and IV sleep all decrease, an important point for elderly readers to bear in mind, and one we shall return to later on.)

What Sleep Does for Us

Common sense tells us that sleep must be, at the very least, restorative. Yet, that simple observation has not yet been proven to the satisfaction of scientists. "The fact is," says Dartmouth's Dr. Peter Hauri, a sleep researcher, "from a strictly neurological and physiological viewpoint, there is no objective proof that any restorative or recuperative processes get under way. And yet we all know, subjectively, that sleep makes us feel better—that we feel refreshed by a good night's sleep and feel miserable when we are sleepless."

These are approximations, based on a report in the *Journal of the American Medical Association*, of three different sleep patterns: a normal one, an insomniac's, and an insomniac on large doses of sleeping pills.

Note that the insomniac was awake more, took longer to fall asleep, and spent less time in Stages III and IV and in REM. The drug user never reached Stage III or IV, and had little REM.

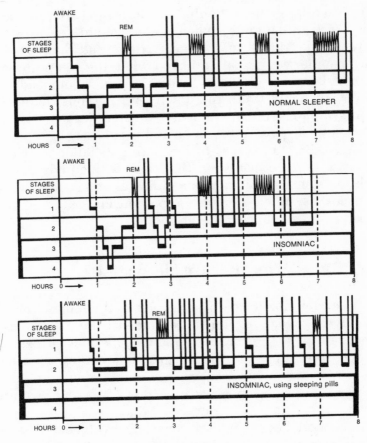

*NREM always precedes REM except in infants, narcoleptics, and those deprived of sleep for 200 or more hours.

While our experience tells us that sleep restores vigor to the body, we now know from research that it does more than merely relieve ordinary physical fatigue. Writes Dr. William C. Dement, one of the pioneer researchers on the subject: "While it is true that muscular fatigue will be ameliorated while the body is 'at rest' during the night, it seems clear that the reversal of fatigue is not the specific function of sleep or the sole reason for its existence."

The elimination of waste products, respite from emotional tension, resynthesis of brain tissue, the cathartic purging of psychic stress—all have been suggested as the reasons for sleep's obvious importance.

Studies on the clinical effects of sleep therapies have revealed that hospital patients showed faster recuperation when allowed as much sleep as they wanted. Children who were two or three years behind the normal rate of progress in school quickly caught up when encouraged to sleep any time they felt like doing so. Chronic fatigue and depression in older people was quickly relieved when the sleep time was increased. And a group of women, all of whom had complained of being tired, run-down, and nervous, found that their symptoms either vanished or significantly lessened after a few days of longer sleep and regular naps.

According to a survey by Dr. Philip M. Tiller, Jr., women who had no more than seven hours of sleep a night had five times as much tension, seven times as much fatigue, and 12 times as much nervous apprehension as their counterparts who slept at least eight hours.

Why Must We Sleep at All?

Theories about the reasons for sleep range from the obvious to the bizarre. Some postulate that sleep first arose as a mechanism for restoration following periods of exertion. Like any machine, the theory goes, our bodies need occasional rest and maintenance, so we shut down at regular intervals. So sleep persisted in the course of evolution because it had important survival value.

A related theory contends that sleep evolved as a preventive device meant to forestall fatigue during subsequent periods of exertion. Others hold that sleep did not evolve at all; it was always there, an important and fundamental feature of nature's orderly, rhythmic ways, as basic as eating.

Other theories are more imaginative and intriguing, but a bit hard to accept. For example, some anthropologically oriented theorists claim that sleep patterns arose because predators had nothing to do at those times of day when their prey was, for one reason or another, impossible to catch. So sleep was relegated to times when hunting would be unprofitable. This, of course, doesn't say *why* we sleep.

A parallel theory states that our early ancestors would have been ill equipped to protect themselves when foraging about in the dark. Since it was in the interest of self-preservation to be cut off from stimulation during those dangerous hours, they invented sleep.

Those with a psychoanalytic bent have their ideas too. Wrote Sigmund Freud, "Somatically, sleep is an act which reproduces intrauterine existence, fulfilling the conditions of repose, warmth, and absence of stimulus." The famous return to the womb. While Freud did not contend that the above analysis identified the *only* reason for sleep, some of his orthodox followers have gone that far, or quite nearly so, and have stretched the master's logic beyond reason.

Perhaps because of our fascination with the content of dreams, the REM state has aroused the greatest speculation. Some say that REM provides a necessary period of stimulation for the brain, which might otherwise atrophy from the absence of stimulation over long periods of time. Psychoanalytic theorists, as everyone knows, have elaborate theories regarding the working out of repressed impulses, desires, and emotions, and have made an art of analyzing the content of dreams.

Dr. Chester Pearlman believes that REM sleep is essential for consolidating memory and for assimilating traumatic experiences encountered during the day. In either case, new information is consolidated and incorporated into one's psychic makeup during REM.

Psychologist Peter Hauri of Dartmouth, agrees: "The function of dreaming is, in a loose sense . . . that of going over what happened during the day. We incorporate whatever has been acquired into the old stores of information, while throwing out the 'garbage,' getting rid of those things we don't really need to retain."

Many of the REM theories were generated by the finding, some time ago, that REM sleep increases after stress, worry, or new learning situations. Professor Ernest Hartmann, a leading sleep researcher, postulates a physiological basis for these observations. He contends that the efficiency of the synapses—microscopic areas between brain cells where impulses are transmitted from one cell to another—is restored during REM. He feels that the structural, enzymatic, and hormonal proteins produced during NREM are used for that purpose.

The speculations and the contending theories—and there are more than the ones we mentioned—are just beginning to penetrate the mysteries of sleep. They are fascinating, and they are promising. But they are still a long way from satisfying the rigorous demands of science. Somehow, the simplest things in nature are often the least amenable to the complexities of experimentation. The interested layman should keep an eye on the new developments, but continue to think of sleep in the usual common sense way—as something we need and need in an efficient and natural form.

Until science can improve on them, we will enjoy the definitions of the poets:

> Sleep, that knits up the ravell'd sleave of care,
> The death of each day's life, sore labour's bath,
> Balm of hurt minds, great nature's second course,
> Chief nourisher in life's feast.
>
> —Shakespeare (*Macbeth*)

The Effects of Sleep Deprivation

In 1895, Lord Rosebery, then Prime Minister of England, resigned his office because of his chronic insomnia. In 1903 he wrote: 'I cannot forget 1895. To lie, night after night, staring wide awake, hopeless of sleep, tormented in nerves, and to realize all that was going on, when I was present, so to speak, like a disembodied spirit, to watch one's own corpse, as it were, day after day, is an experience which no sane man with a conscience would repeat."

The unfortunate gentleman discovered what too many of us have learned—when you don't sleep well you suffer.

Clinical precision may be lacking as to *why* we sleep, but

SYMPTOMS OF SLEEP DEPRIVATION

—Perception deteriorates (resulting in hallucinations, if sleep loss is prolonged).

—Reaction time is damaged (interestingly, studies show that speed of reaction does not simply slow down, as one might expect, but becomes increasingly more erratic and unpredictable, surely a greater hazard than a predictable loss of speed).

—Performance of all tasks is impaired.

—Energy level decreases.

—Motivation diminishes.

—Vulnerability to pain increases.

—Memory becomes faulty.

—Efficiency is impaired.

—Attentiveness is reduced.

—Judgment breaks down.

—Psychologically, one is apt to become negative, listless, hostile, disinterested, depressed.

a good deal is known about what happens to those who do not get enough of it.

Naturally, these ill effects of sleep deprivation vary from one person to another; age, physical condition, emotional well-being, and attitude, all contribute to the differences. The effects will also fluctuate for each person, depending on the circumstances. Sleep loss brought on by unusually stressful situations is more likely to produce severe consequences than sleep loss incurred through, say, careless overeating or travel.

To our list of scientifically proven effects of sleep loss, you can probably add your own symptoms, such as burning eyes, wobbly knees, or loss of appetite. You will doubtless recall everyday mishaps, disasters and catastrophes linked to sleeplessness; car accidents are a common result (studies in both Oklahoma and California revealed that about 20 percent of highway accidents involved sleepy drivers). Think of the loss of confidence and self-esteem, the breakdown of marriages and friendships, and regrettable misjudgments of all kinds, all traceable to unfulfilled sleep needs.

The reader no doubt also knows the psychological difficulties to which the insomniac is heir. You can't help feeling like a freak as you lie there unable to do what comes effortlessly to everyone else. "I feel injured by my insomnia," reported an anonymous sufferer, "as though I have been left out of a marvelous party everyone else enjoys and I can only watch."

Writes another, quoted in Luce and Segal's *Insomnia:* "What hurts most about not being able to sleep is the loneliness. There you are, all alone with yourself while the rest of the world sleeps. There is nothing to distract you from your thoughts, no street noises, no TV. You're faced with yourself. There's no one who cares—no one who *can* care. Everybody's asleep but you."

Most of our knowledge of sleep deprivation has been derived by researchers who systematically aroused people during various stages of sleep.

Of all the stages of sleep, the REM stage, and to a lesser extent, Stage IV, are the ones we can least afford to do without. Generally speaking, a little loss of sleep here and there is compensated for easily and quickly, particularly if the loss was of Stages I, II, or III. Extensive deprivation of Stage IV often results in overall lethargy, with the effects becoming more pronounced as the loss is prolonged.

Early experiments found that even a small amount of deprivation of REM can lead to impairment of learning, memory, and the ability to focus. With extended loss, serious behavioral and psychological disturbances seemed to result. Subjects became confused, muddled, and found even simple tasks difficult to deal with. Eventually, it was felt, REM loss would lead to mental breakdown.

Recent evidence indicates that REM deprivation may not be devastating as once believed. Depressed people, for example, often seem to do better without REM sleep. And many people have been found to function adequately over extended periods of time even when REM was suppressed. Nonetheless, the overall picture is one of increasing disability the longer a person is subjected to REM deprivation.

The studies on REM loss, of course, were done under laboratory conditions, and thus the observed effects are radical. The average insomniac is hardly likely to suffer such extremes. As Dr. Charles Pollack, a prominent sleep specialist points out, "Insomnia is not the same as being deprived of sleep in a laboratory." But the studies provide us with a useful framework for understanding what happens as a result of even mild loss of sleep. And they help explain why persons deprived of sleep will invariably have remarkably vivid dreams and more of them, once they do sleep. Apparently, we need the REM stage so much that when we miss out on some we tend to spend a greater percentage of our subsequent sleep time in that stage. Called compensatory dreaming or REM rebound, this proven fact points up the importance of the REM stage, and is a significant argument against the use of sleeping pills. Drugs inhibit the REM stage of sleep.

As yet there is no evidence of permanent physical damage caused by prolonged sleep loss, although that possibility certainly cannot be discounted. Some scientists suspect that long-range damage may be done to the brain. However, we know so little about the brain, particularly its higher intellectual functions, that it will probably be some time before the question is settled.

Awake for 200 Hours

In a well-publicized "wakathon" for charity, a New York disc jockey named Peter Tripp stayed awake for 200 hours, continuing his regular broadcasts from a glass-enclosed booth in Times Square, and submitting to medical research throughout. After some time of this enforced wakefulness, Tripp began to hallucinate. A series of bizarre delusions culminated with his running naked down a hallway attempting to escape from the doctors, who, he believed, were undertakers attempting to bury him alive. He also reported a prolonged bout with depression subsequent to his vigil.

But Mr. Tripp, of course, was hardly a typical insomniac. Most of us, even on our worst nights, manage to get *some* sleep, and are hardly likely to go more than a few days without some relief. What was remarkable about Mr. Tripp's case and others like his, was that after a solid night's sleep, he was functioning amazingly well. For the average insomniac, recovery of normal functioning is remarkably quick. Even in severe cases, a period of erratic moods, plus extra time needed in compensatory sleep, are usually all the recovering individual has to contend with.

Said one sleep expert, "Given a fair chance, the living body is naturally self-regulating and will tend to make good some temporary loss of sleep now and then by more sleep subsequently, so that on balance it gets as much natural sleep as it needs."

One last word on the effects of sleep loss. The authors have discovered a perplexing incongruity that we have labelled the Insomnia Paradox. Sleep loss is horrible, as any victim will tell you. Realizing that fact will help all of us do what we can to insure that we sleep well. But there is another side to the coin. If you pay *too* much attention to your sleep, or to the possible consequences of losing some, you are likely to worry about it. The result? You will lose sleep!

Dealing with the Insomnia Paradox is a delicate matter. It requires dealing with your own mind carefully. Be concerned, but don't worry. Be aware of the problem, but don't belabor it. Sure, even the loss of a few hours sleep can ruin a day, or worse. But it is probably not as bad as you think.

In chapter four we will discuss the proper attitude to adopt and give you some facts that will help you see the less gloomy side of insomnia. For now it is enough to remind you that insomnia can be easily and naturally overcome. Rest assured that, armed with the knowledge in this book, you will be able to take advantage of W. C. Field's time-tested remedy for insomnia: "Get plenty of sleep!"

What Causes Insomnia?

Mark Twain was a cantankerous insomniac. Once, the author found himself at a friend's home, unable to sleep. The problem was not a new one to Twain, yet he convinced himself that the reason for his failure to sleep was the poor ventilation in the unfamiliar room. He tossed and turned for some time, cursing the stuffy atmosphere. Finally, in a fit of anger, he picked up his shoe and hurled it through the darkness at the window, which he had been unable to open in the conventional way. He heard the sound of shattering glass, inhaled deeply and thankfully, and fell fast asleep. In the morning the well-rested humorist noticed that the glass-enclosed bookcase had been smashed. The window was still locked and intact.

The story has a multitude of lessons for the insomniac, not the least of which is that the mind can play tricks on us. The causes we ascribe to our sleep problems may not be the real ones.

It could well be that your sleep difficulties are attributable to something as simple as the ventilation in your room, or to the humidity, noise, type of mattress, or what you ate for supper. Such factors will be discussed in later chapters, for they definitely affect your sleep, no matter what other elements are involved. In addition to environmental factors, situational ones also affect sleep. Everyone has experienced temporary sleep loss due to some obvious cause—jet lag, an unfamiliar bed, grief over the loss of a loved one, pressure on the job, and so forth. The information in this book will help you find relief until the situation changes and normal sleep resumes.

But if you lose sleep chronically, if you often awaken unrefreshed and are fatigued during the day, it might be a big mistake to attribute your problem only to the situation or the environment. Yet, as Mr. Twain's case reveals, even the most intelligent among us find it more palatable to point the finger of blame at something outside themselves. We seek safe, nonthreatening explanations. They are easier to live with. Unfortunately, with insomnia, they usually cover up the real problems.

Failure to sleep properly is a strange and bewildering phenomenon. Unlike the failure to run fast, write well, multiply, or bake bread, it can't be attributed to lack of skill, poor education, or insufficient talent. Everyone can sleep. Babies are terrific at it. Even dumb beasts can sleep.

If you have any doubt that it should require no great skill, no talent, no artifacts or contrivances to be able to fall asleep and stay there, ask one of your deep-sleeping friends to describe how he or she does it. More than likely the person will be dumbfounded. "What do you mean, how do I go to sleep? I just do. I lie down, close my eyes, and, if I'm sleepy, I just fall asleep. That's all!"

Falling is actually an apt word for it. Like actual falling, it happens without effort or intention, just by creating a situation in which natural principles can take over. The person who wants to sleep well must, like someone who wants to fall, just create a suitable situation and let go.

In her goodness, nature has made it easier to fall asleep than it is to eat. To sleep you don't need to hunt, forage, till, reap, trade, or manufacture. Indeed, that indicates just how vital sleep is—we can go without food much longer than we can go without sleep, and all we lose by doing so is some weight.

Perhaps only breathing requires less effort than falling asleep. We don't do it; it does us. We don't go to sleep so much as sleep comes to us. We don't have to search for it—at best we coax it. Nature does all the work. It is as if our nervous systems were automatic transmissions, capable of shifting into the proper gear—waking, or the several stages of sleep—as and when they are needed.

Then why doesn't it happen?

There is no simple answer. We asked every expert we could, and consulted the rest through the literature. A myriad factors are involved, and the experts often disagree on which are the most important. Insomnia is not a disease, traceable to a germ or an injury. Rather, it is a *sign*, but one that can indicate one or many of a variety of things. About the best generalization we can offer is that chronic insomniacs are somehow out of whack with the rhythms that nature implanted in us.

In addition, the problem may involve an internal desynchronization, with two or more biorhythms fluctuating in periodicities that are incompatible with one another. The nervous system cannot shift gears at the proper time.

Just why is difficult to guess without a detailed knowledge of the individual case. Says Dr. Peter Hauri, "There might be one of a hundred things wrong with a person who can't fall asleep."

With few exceptions, insomnia is a multifaceted problem, involving many aspects of our lives, interrelating and overlapping so much as to make any attempt at identifying one single cause arbitrary and somewhat ludicrous. Everything we experience affects our nervous systems and therefore our sleep.

Of course, certain factors have a definite, often predictable and measurable influence on sleep. Sleep experts are trying to identify those with mathematical precision. Those factors that are known to affect sleep will be discussed in the context of the treatments that are designed to offset them. In this way, our attention will remain where it is most practical—on solutions rather than problems. Here we will give an overview that will provide you with a perspective on the state of the art today. It should convince you that the only way to think of your sleep is holistically.

Broadly speaking, there are three categories of causes: physical, mental, and behavioral/situational. The physicians and psychologists who work with sleep disorders take into account the latter, but treat it with relative lack of seriousness. To their credit, few experts claim to have the answers. They recognize that their specialty is in its infancy and that much research is needed. Indeed, most clinics work in teams, with several disciplines represented.

Unfortunately, one rarely finds nutritionists or other nature-oriented experts on these teams. Most of the thinking tends to run along the usual lines of physical and psychological pathologies. Understandably, the people involved view the problem through the narrow perspective of their own specialties.

We found that there is tremendous disagreement among them—a good-natured disagreement, typified by laudable humility, but one that is revealing. One sleep expert, a psychiatrist, estimates that 85 percent of all insomnia is due to psychiatric causes. Another psychiatrist claims that 60 percent of his patients with insomnia have psychological problems. This is not surprising, when you note that a standard psychological reference defines insomnia as "an anxiety syndrome peculiar to the neurotic personality pattern engendered by civilized society."

By contrast, another sleep clinician—a neurologist—estimates that emotional problems are the cause of insomnia in only 30 percent of his patients. A physiologist feels that one-third are due to psychological causes and that hidden neurological disorders cause, or aggravate, most chronic sleep troubles.

In an article in the *New England Journal of Medicine* two psychiatrists traced sleep problems to psychological factors and advocated the use of medicine and psychotherapy as preferred treatments. In a subsequent issue, a doctor from the National Institute of Health responded: "We cannot agree with their interpretation that psychiatric disturbances are necessarily the cause of insomnia. On the basis of their data, and that of other sleep researchers, there are at least two other interpretations, one being that the chronic sleep deprivation ... may be the cause of the insomniac patient's psychologic disturbances. The other interpretation is that the disturbed psychologic and sleep patterns may be dual manifestations of a more fundamental disorder of physiologic activating or arousal mechanism."

In other, less technical terms, it is impossible to determine whether mental, physical, or other factors are the prime villains. The mind and body affect each other in a circular way. It is as hard to determine which comes first as it is with chickens and eggs. What is interesting about the experts' opinions is that they reflect their fields of expertise, even when it comes to making estimates about percentages.

Trying to Pin It Down

The controversy cannot be resolved now. As the letter quoted above concluded, there is a need for continued research that would "help to elucidate the cause-and-effect relation between the psychologic and sleep disturbances as well as the long-term therapeutic value of nonpharmacologic, nontraditional psychotherapeutic treatment approaches in chronic insomnia."

It must be remembered that we are complex organisms. We are made of myriad parts, the interraction of which all goes to make up the person we call "I." Some parts affect the whole more significantly than others, but we cannot be narrow visioned when it comes to our sleep.

The specialists are, by necessity, narrow visioned. In an age that is so complex that specialists find it difficult to keep up with their own fields, this is inevitable. But we can't help but lament the loss of generalists, and hope that the trend toward natural treatments and holistic health will soon spread to the hospitals and laboratories where they are most conspicuously absent.

Until then, the insomniac who wants to pin down his or

her sleep-depriving factors is likely to encounter the same bewildering situation that a friend of ours named Elliot Cummings faced. A real estate broker whose business had suffered a major setback, Mr. Cummings had been losing sleep for a long time. He saw his family physician, and was given a prescription for sleeping pills. He did not like the side effects, gave the pills up, but did not know where to turn. A friend recommended a psychoanalyst. The analyst, a strict Freudian, told our friend that his insomnia was probably "an unconscious fear of being attacked while in a defenseless position." When our friend suggested that the explanation was far fetched, he was offered an alternative diagnosis—he might be afraid he would walk in his sleep and attack other people.

He cancelled his therapy and visited another physician. This one hypothesized that our friend was not metabolizing serotonin effectively (serotonin is a brain chemical linked with the onset of sleep). Verifying his diagnosis, however, involved a costly series of visits to a sleep clinic, which was, to my friend, out of the question.

He continued to survey those in the know. A nutritionist told him he had vitamin deficiencies and poor digestion, and prescribed a new diet and a plethora of supplements. Others—amateur sleuths and health nuts—suggested all kinds of causes and all kinds of solutions, of which there are as many combinations as there are sheep to count. Bewildered, Mr. Cummings complained about his inability to come to terms with all the suggested causes. The person to whom he was speaking offered this unintentionally brilliant reply: sleep on it!

Eventually, Cummings conquered his insomnia by employing a variety of treatments. Just which ones worked for this particular man is irrelevant here, since solutions vary from one person to the next. Mr. Cummings' story, however, should drive home the one point that every person concerned with the reasons for poor sleep should keep in mind: Do not view your sleep troubles as aberrant from the rest of your 24-hour day or from your entire mental, physical, and emotional condition. This may seem obvious, but you would be surprised how many people refuse to accept it. Luce and Segal report: "Since sleep is inextricably interknit with a person's general health and way of life, it is unreasonable and illogical to expect good sleep during an inherently unhealthy life. Nonetheless, this is the expectation of most people."

Look for ways to improve your life as a whole. In doing so you will find yourself sleeping more soundly. In seeking the specific roots of your sleep problem, weigh all the factors. Be vigilant about it. And, in your search for solutions, be open minded. Just as you can move a table by pulling on any of its legs, you can improve your sleep by dealing with any area of your life: physical, mental, nutritional, behavioral, or situational. As yet, there are no universal palliatives, no guaranteed, instant cures. But, as we shall soon see, there is a veritable supermarket of effective, natural procedures to choose from without resorting to drugs.

CHAPTER THREE

THE CASE
AGAINST DRUGS

Not poppy, nor mandragora,
Nor all the drowsy syrups of the world,
Shall ever medicine thee to that sweet sleep,
Which thou owedst yesterday.
     —Shakespeare (*Othello*)

Steven Friedland, an insomniac musician, tells the following story of his experience with sleeping pills:

"I had always been one of those whose sleep became disturbed during a crisis or an emotional upset. In 1968 I went through a particularly turbulent period that resulted in a prolonged bout with insomnia. After a few days a friend said, Why don't you take something for it?—the classic modern response to any physical problem.

"Recalling the TV commercials where tension-ridden nonsleepers were suddenly transformed into serene Buddhas sleeping with the ease of newborn pups, I bought some sleeping pills at my friendly pharmacy. On the first night, I took the recommended dosage, but still could not get to sleep quickly enough to satisfy my longing. I upped the dose, convinced that, since I had obtained the drug without a prescription, it could not be terribly dangerous.

"For the next three nights, I continued with my arbitrarily high dosage, and sure enough, I fell asleep fairly quickly. I did not feel especially good during the days, but one seldom does during a period as stressful as the one I was in. On the fourth night the pills did not work. Thinking I must be exceptionally tense, I sweated it out. When, a few hours later, sleep still had not come, I took some extra pills. I fell asleep, but the next day I was nauseous, dull, somewhat more irritable than usual.

"Alarmed that I had to so greatly exceed the recommended dosage before the pills would work, I decided to see a physician to get the *real thing*, a prescribed sleeper. I got it with no trouble whatsoever.

'What's your problem?' the doctor asked.

'I can't sleep.'

'How long has this persisted?'

'About a week.'

'What have you been taking for it?'

"That was all he asked. He was habituated into thinking along rigidly allopathic lines: for problem X, prescribe drug Y. I could see his mind linking symptom to chemical, as though he were taking a matching test in medical school.

"The drug he prescribed was a knockout. I fell asleep quickly every night for a week. I stopped passing my daytime hours worrying about whether I would fall asleep that night. As far as my indigestion, dullness, and lethargy were concerned, I attributed them to my still unresolved crisis, and my previous lack of sleep. Then one night the pills didn't work. I attributed it to chance, suffered through an erratic night and a dismal day. Next night, it happened again. Angry, worried about what appeared to be a relapse of insomnia, I took an extra pill. That did the trick. The next night I didn't even bother starting out with the original quantity. On the phone, the doctor okayed my decision.

"Once again, sleep came easily. But, I had fallen prone to fits of depression, my stomach was chronically upset, I had lost a once voracious appetite, I would incur sudden fits of the chills, and my mind was alarmingly dull and disoriented. Oddly, the crisis that had precipitated my insomnia had pretty much been resolved. There was no reason for me to be so miserable. I had even cured my insomnia, with a little help from my pills.

"By a stroke of luck for which I shall remain eternally grateful, I happened to mention all this to a friend whom I considered, at the time, a back-to-nature freak. He immediately suspected my medication. I defended my pills like a knight in shining armor. My friend, however, was unrelenting. He predicted that, if I continued to rely on sleeping pills, my insomnia would soon return. I called him a misguided radical, popped my pills defiantly, and went to bed.

"It took over an hour to fall asleep. I blamed it on the agitation caused by my friend's argument. The next night and the one following, it took even longer to fall asleep. I considered upping my dosage again. Then my friend's warning—that there was no end to raising the dosage—came to mind. Maybe he was right to warn of my becoming dependent; maybe he was right too about my pills being responsible for all my new daytime maladies.

"I stopped taking the pills. That night I couldn't sleep. Nor the next. What sleep I did manage to get was restless, percolating with wild nightmares. During the day, my previous symptoms—especially the nausea and weakness—intensified. I had difficulty catching my breath at times. Then I began to twitch involuntarily.

"Blaming it all on the relapse of insomnia, I began to regret having forsaken my faithful pills. I told my friend that I intended to reunite with them. He called me a junkie. He was right. I had become physically and psychologically dependent on drugs. He recommended a doctor who was inclined toward drugless remedies. The doctor put me on a smaller dose of the pills, then continued to decrease the dosage gradually over the period of a month. At times the withdrawal process was absolute hell. But eventually I was myself again. My frightful symptoms disappeared, and I slept soundly once again."

The story is a typical one. Sleep medication almost invariably sets a pattern in motion: tolerance, increased dosage, tolerance, another increase in dosage, psychological dependence, physical addiction, devastating side effects, severe withdrawal symptoms (if the person is lucky enough to be told to stop taking the pills). And the sad irony is that sleeping pills do not cure insomnia. Indeed, they are a perfect example of the remedy being more lethal than the malady it is designed to cure.

The Prevalence of Drug Use

An estimated 20 million Americans take barbiturates, the most commonly used form of "sleeper," and another 30 million take tranquilizers regularly. Collectively, we consume about 600 *tons* of sleeping pills a year—about 30 million doses a night. Forty million prescriptions for sleepers are filled annually.

One doctor estimates that there are enough sleeping pills produced in this country each year to put every man, woman, and child in the United States to sleep, artificially, for 200 hours. When added to the amount of money spent on non-prescribed medication, the total is staggering. Estimates range from 100 million to 175 million dollars annually—a huge drain on the budgets of harried families, and a windfall indeed for the pharmaceutical industry. Sleepers are second in sales only to aspirin.

As of April, 1976, there were over 200 brands of sleeping pills on the market with research under way for 39 more. The think tanks and laboratories are ever brewing up new concoctions to tranquilize, sedate, or conversely, to speed up our stressed citizens, who are accustomed to taking a pill for whatever ails them. Yet, according to a task force at the department of Health, Education and Welfare, the overwhelming majority of new drugs are only slight variations on already existing ones. They are reportedly being developed for the sole purpose of obtaining patents for the inventing companies.

Recently, hope has come from Washington. In 1962 an amendment by the late Senator Kefauver provided that sleep-aids and sedatives must be shown, by substantial evidence, to be safe and effective for their claimed uses. According to Senator Gaylord Nelson in 1977, "The manufacturers have had 15 years to produce the evidence but they have failed to do so."

Senator Nelson chaired a subcommittee whose purpose was to investigate these drugs. Its expert witnesses—almost all M.D.'s—testified overwhelmingly that over-the-counter sleeping pills were dangerous and ineffective. "My feeling is the over-the-counter sleep drugs should not be sold," said Dr. Anthony Kales in an interview in the *Medical World*

News, "The use and availability of these drugs is not to the advantage of the average patient."

Dr. Kales' remark is a common one among sleep experts, and an increasingly common one among physicians in general. In most cases the mistrust of drugs extends to prescribed, as well as over-the-counter varieties.

Part of the problem has been that physicians have not had complete information on sedatives, tranquilizers, barbiturates, and other medicines that cross their desks. This is due to inadequate testing, incomplete labelling, and misleading promotional literature. Research on the effects of drugs tends to limit itself to the effects of, at most, one to three days of use. Hardly any attention has been given to the longer-range effects, despite the fact that over half of all the prescriptions for sleepers are given for periods of three months or more.

The doctor's usual source of information on drugs is the *Physician's Desk Reference*, which consists of nothing more than the package inserts produced by the drug manufacturers themselves. The *Reference* is, really, a form of advertising. Many of the drugs are labelled "nonhabit forming," "safe," or "effective." When investigated, such claims have more often than not turned out to be exaggerated or untrue. At best, the drugs are "safe and effective" for a few days.

The statistics lead to the nearly inescapable conclusion that we have been careless about public safety. In the fiscal year 1974-75, the pharmaceutical industry recorded sales of seven billion dollars. That figure could simply reflect the alarming degree to which Americans gobble up medication. But this figure is more revealing: the drug companies spent one billion dollars on promotion—four times the amount spent on research! About one-third of that promotion budget was spent peddling pharmaceutical wares to doctors.

The Side Effects

Sleeping pills can cause more serious disorders than the sleeplessness they are designed to correct. According to Dr. Malcolm Lader, "All sleeping pills affect persons adversely for a minimum of 18 hours." Here is how:

```
┌─────────────────────────────────────────────────────────┐
│                                                         │
│   KNOWN SIDE EFFECTS OF SLEEPING PILLS                  │
│   –impaired digestion                                   │
│   –circulation disorders                                │
│   –blood deterioration                                  │
│   –respiratory problems                                 │
│   –blurred vision                                       │
│   –loss of appetite (anorexia)                          │
│   –skin rashes                                          │
│   –high blood pressure                                  │
│   –lowered resistance to colds and infection (some pills contain │
│     ingredients known to destroy white blood corpuscles) │
│   –dermatitis                                           │
│   –kidney and liver ailments                            │
│   –central nervous system damage (dulling the brain)    │
│   –impaired memory                                      │
│   –dizziness                                            │
│   –irritability                                         │
│   –confusion                                            │
│   –lack of coordination                                 │
│   –anxiety                                              │
│   –depression                                           │
│                                                         │
└─────────────────────────────────────────────────────────┘
```

Obviously, there are many kinds of sleeping pills, and the effects vary from one to another and from one person to another. The above list was compiled without distinguishing between the various drugs and their ingredients. More details can be obtained by consulting the Appendix, where you will find a run-down on the ten most frequently used prescription drugs.

The harmful side effects of "sleepers" are not limited to the powerful prescription drugs. Tens of millions of people make the tragic mistake of thinking that, if a drug can be purchased without a prescription, it must be safe. Highly advertised sleeping pills, like Nytol, Dormin, Sleep-eze, and Sominex are dangerous. They contain as their main sedative ingredient an antihistamine, usually methapyrilene, known by the trade name, Histadyl.

A well-known pharmacological textbook, authored by Drs. Goodman and Gilman, lists the following among the potential side effects of antihistamines: dizziness, incoordination, blurred vision, nervousness, anorexia, frequent urination, skin rashes, and sometimes blood changes. And, while antihistamines will make a person dangerously drowsy, they do not appear to help actual sleep. Reported Dr. Sumner M. Kalman to the Senate subcommittee, "We found few careful studies in the submissions given to us by manufacturers, and we had to . . . look into the scientific literature to find out if there were controlled studies where antihistamines had been given alone. We found evidence that higher doses, not the doses usually used in over-the-counter preparations, could help a person to fall asleep. But there wasn't very much evidence."

Scopolamine and bromides, perhaps the most common sleeping pill ingredients, were both found toxic by a government study panel, which urged that they be banned. Of bromides, a 1975 Food and Drug Administration panel said, "The effective dose differs little from the poisonous dose." The FDA also noted that some patients who had taken too much scopolamine had been committed to psychiatric institutions with "a mistaken diagnosis of schizophrenia."

Dr. Kalman's testimony had this to say about bromides: "The bromides were found too dangerous for over-the-counter use because of their tendency to accumulate when used chronically and, by accumulation in the body to pose a serious hazard to health. . . . The curious way by which bromides work—the displacement of the normal chloride ion in the body by the bromide ion so that a central nervous system depression is achieved—makes the use of these agents totally unsuitable for over-the-counter use. It is not rational for *occasional* use."

These two case studies, cited by Dr. Julius Rice in *Ups and Downs*, are typical of the frightening side effects of "sleepers," effects that the user rarely anticipates:

"A woman who spent 30 years of her life fearing mental illness because her father had been hospitalized for depression when he was a young man, was a willing and regular recipient of anything that "calmed nerves" and accordingly a frequent visitor to her family physician and to the neighborhood pharmacy. The druggist, always an obliging collaborator, gave her all the Sominex she wanted when she 'fell out' with her doctor . . . She began 'seeing things.' In spite of insistent questioning, she denied taking drugs. Arrangements for her hospitalization were already made when a search of the bathroom revealed the abundant Sominex concealed in a drawer. She meekly protested that she 'just had to sleep.' She was told by the pharmacist that Sominex was a mild sedative, which would not harm her."

The second case is of a 22-year-old graduate student who "flipped out" a month before graduation. "He had had more trouble than usual sleeping, had been unable to study, and for a few days prior to his homecoming had seen 'weird things.' He felt that he had been 'grinding' too hard. The college psychologist and physician concurred with his clinical assessment. His family physician referred him for psychiatric consultation after an extensive 'physical workup' had failed to reveal an organic basis for the complaints."

Interestingly, the young man had been his old self as soon as he came home. He attributed this to the respite from the grind of school. It turned out that the improvement was due to his no longer taking Sleep-Eze. He had taken the drug for the three days prior to his breakdown, because a pharmacist recommended it for his temporary insomnia. He said that the medicine—which he had taken each of three nights in above average dosages—had not helped him sleep.

Each year, thousands of people die from the use of sleeping pills. The National Institute of Mental Health estimates that one-third of those deaths were not suicides. The victims die unwittingly when they carelessly have a few cocktails and soon afterwards pop their pill to go to sleep. Alcohol and soporific drugs, especially barbiturates, do not mix.

Some of the deaths occur on the road, where overly sedated drivers are truly a menace. It is estimated that drug users of all kinds are involved in about 15,000 traffic deaths a year. A study determined that drug users have ten times as many accidents as do nonusers, and that one out of every 12 drivers is under the influence of sleeping pills or amphetamines.

Another cause of death stems from the fact that your body's tolerance for the drug varies tremendously from one moment to the next, depending on your physical condition, food intake, the presence of other drugs, and several other factors. The variation is so wide and so unpredictable that a small dose, sufficient to put you to sleep one day, might kill you the next.

Having a prescription filled, swallowing a pill or two, or three, to relieve the torment of sleeplessness, hardly seems as ominous, or as socially unacceptable, as injecting a hypodermic needle filled with heroin. Yet it can be equally devastating.

Sleeping Pills Are Addictive

Addiction begins when the initial dosage is no longer effective in bringing on sleep. Virtually every drug tested has been shown to lose its effectiveness within two weeks (the exception, reportedly, is Dalmane, or Flurazepam, which maintains effectiveness for three to four weeks). The reason for this is that the user's body develops a tolerance for the drug, as it might for any toxic agent.

According to one expert, "We have concluded that drug dependency will develop in any medication . . . that shows a rapid development of tolerance to its sleep inducing effects. The same principle applies to alcoholic beverages, popularly used as sleep medication."

With over-the-counter drugs the situation is particularly delicate, since they are usually not very effective in the dosage recommended on the packages. Desperate for sleep, insomniacs tend to disregard common sense and sound advice, raising the dosage arbitrarily. And, because they can buy as much of the product as they want, whenever they want, there are no sanctions.

Eventually, higher and higher doses are required to bring on sleep, the side effects become increasingly severe, and the users become sleeping pill junkies. Commonly, the addicted persons will take amphetamines during the day to counteract the dullness and fatigue brought on by last night's sleeping pills. In so doing they are running the risk of having drugs dominate their entire lives, and the chances of serious, perhaps fatal consequences rise sharply.

The situation is compounded further by the users' belief that the pills are actually helping them, long after their actual effectiveness has worn off. "The individual may, because he *believes* the drug is putting him to sleep, actually be able to relax enough so that he can doze off," states Dr. Peter Hauri, "But the pill itself isn't doing a thing. On the contrary, the pills are most probably going to disturb the pattern of his sleep, and his sleep is certainly going to be far more rotten because he's taken them."

We used the word "junkie" knowing full well the socially unacceptable connotations of the word. But it is not an inappropriate one. Says Dr. Harris Isbell, formerly Chief of the Public Health Service Addiction Center in Lexington, Kentucky: "Invariably, the user (of barbiturates or amphetamines) ends up a more socially destructive character than a heroin addict."

If you have been using sleeping pills for some time, and especially if you have increased your dosage, do not take these alarming facts as a signal to stop suddenly. The barbiturate habit is more difficult to break than heroin addiction. The effects of sudden withdrawal can be more dangerous, and more agonizing, than the celebrated "cold turkey" of the hard-core drug addict. The effects may include: extreme anxiety, stomach cramps, nausea, vomiting, weakness, serious weight loss, rapid breathing, fever, hallucinations, dehydration, convulsions, uncontrollable twitching, nightmares, delusions, hypertension, and, of all things, insomnia!

The disruption of sleep caused by the sleeping pill withdrawal is often what makes it difficult for persons to carry through with their withdrawal program. They easily convince themselves that their sleeplessness is simply a recurrence of a disease, much like getting the flu a second time in one winter. They then fall back on the pills as a way to induce sleep again.

Anyone who has become dependent on sleeping medication may need to go through a withdrawal program supervised by doctors. This case study, reported in *Psychology Today* tells the familiar story: "Her chemical dependency called for an 18-month tapering off under careful medical supervision that had to intensify as she worked her dosage down. Even though her final step to drug freedom was very small, our recordings showed that she got no sleep at all on her first night without pills. She then got eight hours of uneven sleep during the next day. For the next three days, her sleep onset came about two hours later each day—as if she were on a [longer than 24-hour day]."

Eventually the patient was back within normal sleep patterns for her age. But it might not have occurred if the doctors had not been vigilant. "Because we anticipated her withdrawal pains, we were able to counter her attempts to use them as new evidence of intractable insomnia and as an excuse to take more hypnotics. In times of distress, such patients have a well-learned impulse to return to the comfort of their drugs."

Dr. Anthony Kales devised a way to detoxify patients without serious complications. He withdraws one clinical dose of the drug (the amount normally taken at night) once every week. The length of time of withdrawal depends, of course, on the amount of medication the person has been using.

Dr. Kales' method seems to be a safe one. If you have been using drugs regularly, it is probably the best way to get off the habit, provided you are determined to do so on your own. The wisest step, however, is to undergo withdrawal under medical supervision. The supervision may last a long time, and cost a lot of money, but the benefits of being drug-*in*dependent are well worth it.

Sleeping Pills Disturb Sleep

A few years ago, Dr. Kales, then director of the Sleep Research and Treatment Center at the Hershey Medical Center in Pennsylvania, reported a startling observation: ten insomniacs who had been using sleeping pills for some time and were continuing to use them, slept as poorly as or worse than a comparable group of insomniacs who were receiving no medication at all. This finding gave rise to a category of illness labelled drug-dependency insomnia—insomnia actually caused by sleeping pills.

A look at how barbiturates, the most frequently used sleep-inducing chemicals, do their work will give us a better idea of why they distort normal sleep, and also why they have harmful, addictive effects. This description is quoted from a pamphlet titled *Sedatives*, published by the U.S. Department of Health, Education, and Welfare:

The principal response elicited by barbiturates is a depression of the central nervous system. They act upon the cerebral centers and interfere with the passage of impulses in the brain. They appear to affect the enzyme processes by which energy is acquired, stored in the protoplasm of the cells, and utilized. They depress brain function, and in large doses depress the brain centers responsible for maintaining the rhythm of respiration.

These drugs, then, do not induce natural sleep; they simply knock you out. The chemical processes of the brain are disrupted to the point where stuporlike unconsciousness is impossible to avoid. As Dr. Edmund Jacobson put it, sleep drugs work by "delivering a knock-out blow to the brain cells. You sleep because your nerve cells are paralyzed by what you swallow." Considering the side effects of drugs, the insomniac might be better off hitting himself over the head with a hammer.

The distinction between natural sleep and drug-induced stupor is well described in this passage from Dr. Herbert Sheldon:

Drugs do not produce sleep. . . . In sleep the body is normally engaged in its most efficient reparative and building processes; in narcosis it is engaged in resisting and throwing off poison. This is the reason that sleep is a process of renewal and recuperation, while narcosis is an exhaustive process. The first conserves energy, the second wastes energy. Following sleep, the muscles are stronger; following narcosis the muscles are weak and tremulous. The will is weakened by narcosis; it is strengthened by sleep. Weakness and paralysis of the nerves follow the use of narcotics; the nerves are renewed and strengthened in sleep. In sleep the heartbeat is regular; in narcosis the heartbeat is irregular, even excited. A night of sleep prepares the digestive organs for the normal performance of their functions; narcosis leaves the digestive organs weak—there is nausea, a furred tongue, loss of appetite, dyspepsia, sometimes jaundice.

Perhaps the most decisive clinical argument against drug-induced sleep is the fact that it severely interferes with the REM, or dreaming stage of sleep. Patients tend to spend a tremendously disproportionate amount of time in compensatory dreaming during their first normal sleep following a drugged sleep. In the case of prolonged drug-induced sleep, a veritable orgy of nightmares ensues. While no one is quite sure why we need the REM stage so much, or what it actually accomplishes, we know enough to say that suppressing it will seriously deter the beneficial influences that arise from natural sleep.

Even the staunchest antidrug crusader would not be terribly opposed to someone's taking a pill once in a great while, if one night's sleep is in question, or if the person is suffering from some unbearable pain. However, any steady pill-taking should really be avoided at all costs, if only because the pills won't work for very long. Says Dr. Peter Hauri, director of the Dartmouth Sleep Laboratory, "All sleeping pills become ineffective after two or three, or at the very outside, four weeks of steady use. After that period of time, they simply don't work."

If You Must

Despite the overwhelming evidence against medication, many people will continue to rely on it. Considering our customary ways of thinking and the reluctance of the medical community to recognize the dangers, the drug industry may not be in serious trouble yet. In fact, dangerous as they are, pills may sometimes be used appropriately. Even Dr. Hauri, an opponent of sleeping pills, is not opposed to their use at certain times.

"If an individual is getting himself all uptight and into some sort of bind about his inability to sleep; and if this should continue for a few nights running, then he might be moving into a vicious cycle. . . . So for myself, if I start getting miserable, I'll take a sleeping pill and that will knock me out. I know, however, that the pill-induced sleep will be lousy, because hypnotic drugs suppress the dreaming phase of sleep. And then, the following night, I would expect something which is called the 'REM rebound:' That is, in the next sleep period I'd be making up for the dreams that were suppressed the night before."

If you feel you must use medication on occasion, follow these important points to minimize the danger:

- Always get a prescription from your doctor. Don't ask a friend to lend you a couple of pills, or plead with your pharmacist for the strongest drug on his shelves.
- Never try to refill a prescription without your doctor's knowledge.
- Ask your doctor what the prescribed drug's side effects are, if there is any danger of addiction, and if it is entirely necessary.
- If he says there is no danger, suspect him of being too cavalier. Offer up the arguments cited here, and if he does not counter them to your satisfaction, see another doctor.
- Learn as much as you can about the drug in question. Consult Goodman and Gilman's, *The Pharmacological Basis of Therapeutics; The Physician's Desk Reference; Pharmacopoeia;* and the descriptions of the ten most popular drugs in the Appendix.
- Never take pills after drinking. You might end up very sick, or very dead.
- Husband and wife should not both take pills on the same night. Someone should be alert, just in case.
- Do not take pills the night before a long drive or a potentially strenuous activity.
- Keep the pills away from your children. If they have trouble sleeping or are hyperactive, see your doctor or psychologist.
- Stay away from over-the-counter drugs. They are not very effective, and are as hazardous as prescribed medication, perhaps more so if used unsupervised.
- The recently popularized benzyodiazepines, such as Valium and Librium, *seem*, at this point, to produce less serious side effects than comparable drugs.
- Of the well-tested "sleepers," some doctors lean toward Flurazepam, or Dalmane. Says Dr. Elliot Weitzman, director of the Sleep-Wake Disorders Unit at Montefiore Hospital, "Flurazepam is quite effective for several weeks. However, there is no knowledge of its effect after more than a month. It apparently does not reduce REM sleep as many other drugs do. But it does reduce Stage III and IV sleep."

In 1976, with the mere prospect of a swine flu epidemic, the nation's minds moved immediately to chemistry, not to nature. We hurriedly manufactured a vaccine and began to administer it, virtually untested. It was a typical response to disease in a drug-oriented world.

That attitude must be replaced with a more congenial relationship with nature if we are to avoid becoming a nation of junkies. Already, in the words of Dr. Quentin Regestein, "this country is awash in a pandemic of hypnotic drug abuse. Six to eight percent of the adult population is taking prescribed hypnotics. Combine this with the legions of people who drink themselves into oblivion, and it appears that America is lying stuporous a little bit after bedtime."

It is time to apply a natural, holistic approach to all disease with a special emphasis on prevention. Therefore, let us leave the gloomy consideration of drugs and discuss the many natural ways to promote sound, natural sleep.

CHAPTER FOUR

YOUR BODY AND YOUR SLEEP

How to Deal With Medical Problems that Affect Sleep

If you have chronic sleep problems, the first thing you should do is determine whether or not medical factors are in any way responsible. Insomnia has been linked clinically with several serious pathologies. This chapter will be brief, because the treatment of serious illness is beyond our scope. Our purpose is, primarily, to make you aware of possible medical causes of insomnia, which you might not otherwise consider. The methods for treating insomnia that are discussed throughout the book will probably help you regardless of the cause of your problem, and might even provide some relief from illness. But be sure to see your doctor or a sleep specialist if you suspect any of the following medical factors are interfering with your sleep.

Asthma sufferers are often awakened by attacks in the night, usually in the earlier stages of sleep. Moderate (not vigorous) afternoon exercise has been recommended because it seems to increase the percentage of time spent in Stages III and IV of sleep. However, this is inconclusive, and is certainly not to be taken as a treatment for the asthma itself. Asthmatics should not take sleeping pills under any circumstances, as they depress the respiratory control centers in the brain, compounding breathing difficulties. In addition to your doctor's advice, the breathing exercises mentioned in a later chapter should help, as should many of the antistress procedures mentioned in chapter five.

Coronary patients are often stricken with attacks of angina pectoris (chest pains) that awaken them during the night. According to one study, about 80 percent of these nighttime attacks occur during REM sleep. While medication is commonly used to treat angina, since it can enlarge the blood vessels, doctors advise against the use of any drugs that suppress REM sleep. That, of course, includes sleeping pills. The REM rebound that occurs subsequent to REM loss may increase the risk of angina attacks in these patients.

Most serious illnesses can, of course, interfere with sleep. We discussed asthma and angina because they are relatively common, and because there was something useful to say about them.

Other medical problems known to contribute to sleep difficulties include ulcers, migraine and cluster headaches, hyperthyroidism, hypothyroidism, arthritis, diabetes, kidney disease, epilepsy, and Parkinson's disease. Naturally, any serious illness is going to affect sleep in some way. The ones mentioned here are known to interfere with sleep directly, and often without the insomniac's realizing it.

Medications As Mysterious Insomnia Inducers

The use of drugs is another sleep-robber that requires medical attention in most cases. Here are three revealing cases. One insomniac we know, an artist named Ed Crane, was wise enough to avoid sleeping pills because he had heard about their side effects. Unfortunately, he was not as discriminating about the amphetamines he was taking to stimulate his tired body into action during the day, nor of the antidepressant drugs he was taking to overcome "the blahs." Like most drug users, he did not realize that the pills he thought would counteract the effects of sleep loss were actually interfering with his sleep. It took a last-resort visit to a sleep specialist to enlighten him.

Then there is the woman we interviewed who suffered insomnia, mysteriously enough, only in late summer and early fall. She was bewildered by this predictable pattern.

Finally, she discovered the reason behind it. A sufferer of severe allergies, she had been in the habit of taking large doses of antihistamines during the hay fever season—late summer and early fall. One year, fed up with the drowsiness that the pills induced, she decided to try doing without them. Her experiment did nothing for her hay fever symptoms which raged on unchecked, but a remarkable thing happened: she began to sleep better.

Confused (after all, why should you sleep better when you *stop* taking a drug that makes you drowsy?) she consulted a doctor. Fortunately, the doctor had done his homework. He knew that antihistamines—like tranquilizers and amphetamines—suppress REM sleep. They lead to the same difficulties that we described in the chapter on sleeping pills.

Karen Elder is a young woman who began to have sleep problems about the time she was married. Disturbed by the coincidence, she wondered if sharing a bed with her husband, or perhaps some deep, unconscious neurosis stirred up by marriage, might be responsible. She got herself so despondent about the latter possibility that she went to a psychologist. Still she did not sleep as well as she once did. Then one day she read a report on the alleged dangers of birth control pills, which she had been taking since her marriage. Concerned, she switched to another contraceptive method. Soon she began sleeping well again. She could not figure out why. It seems that female sex hormones influence the pituitary gland and the sleep center in the brain. The Pill can alter hormonal balance enough to affect sleep— in some cases by causing the woman to sleep more, in others by causing insomnia.

Drugs used in connection with medical problems are usually prescribed by a physician. For that reason, and because these compounds are powerful, patients who suspect that their sleep is being interfered with by such drugs should consult with their doctors before abandoning any medication outright. It should be noted that some physicians are so enamored of the wonders of chemistry that they ignore the mounting evidence against certain drugs. If your physician is not sympathetic to your desire to cut down or eliminate a drug, or if he tosses off as nonsense your suggestion that a medication might be interfering with your sleep, consider seeing another doctor.

In some cases a trade-off will have to be decided upon. If the drug is, in fact, interfering with your sleep (and usually this can only be determined by a doctor or by withdrawing from the drug and seeing how your sleep changes), but is needed for medical purposes, you and your doctor will have to decide whether the loss of sleep is good enough reason to give it up. In some cases the drug can be discontinued in favor of an alternative that does not disturb sleep.

Physiological Conditions That Can Disrupt Sleep: Several forms of pathology that occur during sleep are known to contribute to insomnia. These can usually be diagnosed only in a sleep laboratory. You may go to your regular doctor with complaints of interrupted sleep or constant fatigue but, unless he is familiar with the latest sleep research, he will rarely suspect one of these disorders.

Sleep apnea, according to Dr. Elliot Weitzman, director of Montefiore Hospital's sleep center, "is a syndrome in which patients have abnormal respiratory function during sleep such that they stop breathing." (A more complete description of apneas and all other sleep disorders can be found in the Appendix.)

Found in approximately five percent of the patients who visit sleep clinics, apnea often goes undetected for years. In this affliction, the body's automatic control of breathing breaks down as it shifts from waking to sleep. Sometimes the breathing will cease for as long as a minute. The person awakens with a start and gasps for air with a loud snore.

This can be repeated as many as 400 to 500 times a night. But, the interruptions are usually so brief that the victims are totally unaware of them. All they know is that they do not sleep well, that they are groggy and drowsy all day, and that their families complain about their loud snoring.

Researchers are not in agreement about whether apnea is a cause of insomnia. The illness may be entirely unrelated to "difficulty initiating or maintaining sleep." Doctors at Stanford think apnea does cause insomnia; doctors at Montefiore think it does not. In any event, the disorder is more common than anyone believed a few years ago. Anyone concerned about sleep should be made aware of it.

If that description of apnea sounds familiar, you are well advised to see a doctor, who will either observe your sleep in his office or refer you to a sleep clinic where all-night monitoring can determine whether or not you have apnea. If you are over 40 and if you have a tendency toward obesity, you stand a better chance of having apnea.

At this time, the only successful cure for sleep apnea is rather drastic, a type of tracheotomy—a surgical incision in the windpipe that permits unobstructed breathing during sleep, and is covered during the day.

Nocturnal myoclonus is another insomnia-causing sleep pathology. One study connected myoclonus to 10 to 20 percent of chronic insomnia cases. In this disorder the legs jerk abruptly every 25 to 40 seconds in a periodic manner. Attacks may last for minutes or for several hours. The jerking will arouse the sleeper as many as 400 times a night, but the person may not be aware of the cause.

If your spouse complains of being kicked in the night, if you often have discomfort in your lower leg muscles, or if you have "restless leg syndrome" (an inability to keep your legs still while lying awake), you should see your physician or a sleep specialist for advice. Doctors are still searching for a cure for myoclonus. Some drugs have shown promise, but not to the degree hoped for. Nonetheless, it is important to determine whether or not you have this disorder.

Circadian Rhythm Disturbance is a category of sleep disorder that causes apparent insomnia. Some insomniacs seem to suffer from something roughly analogous to permanent jet-lag. Their biological rhythms are chronically out of phase with their social environments, or their cycles are longer than the normal 24 hours. They might, for example, have cycles that last 25 to 27 hours. After a week, what is still 8:00 P.M. to everyone else can be two o'clock in the morning to them.

These people sleep normally, but at the "wrong times," in relation to the 24-hour day that ordinary social and business conventions require. If they are aware of the nature of the difficulty (most of them are not, for it simply seems to them that frequently they can't get to sleep), and if their professional schedule and family life enable them to sleep and wake at unconventional times, then the problem can be solved easily.

But that is rare. Sleep researchers, newly aware of this problem, are investigating ways to recondition those out-of-whack rhythms. One promising method, related to us by Montefiore's Dr. Weitzman, consists of confining the patient to an environment in which there are no outer stimuli—no windows, clocks, schedules, or other infringements. Once a pattern is recognized, the doctors can then reprogram the person's sleep-wake rhythms by systematically adjusting the time the patient goes to sleep.

The Anti-Sleep Effect of Smoking and Drinking

According to the *Medical Tribune* (November 24, 1969) heavy smokers have a harder time falling asleep, and spend less time in the important Stage IV and REM states than do nonsmokers. Dr. Quentin R. Regestein of the Sleep Clinic at Peter Bent Brigham Hospital, Boston, says that smokers using more than three packs a day are "subject to waking episodes several hours after sleep onset, during which they need a cigarette."

The *Medical Tribune* article further stated that, upon giving up the weed, the persons were able to fall asleep faster, sleep longer with fewer interruptions, and, after a period of compensation, have the normal amount of REM sleep.

If you are a heavy smoker, and particularly if you wake up craving a smoke, it is a good bet that cigarettes contribute to your problem.

How to stop, or at least cut down? As anyone who has tried knows, it is rarely easy. There are many organizations and books that claim success in helping people to stop smoking. The SmokEnders course seems to have been successful in most cases. The group has had more than 30,000 graduates, and claims that only six of every 100 ever smoke again. The course is nine weeks and the sessions are run by SmokEnders graduates. You cut down gradually for five weeks, stop, and then attend four more weeks of meetings for reinforcement. For information write SmokEnders' World, Phillipsburg, New Jersey, 08865.

A reportedly valuable book for anyone who wants to kick the smoking habit is Herbert Brean's, *How to Stop Smoking,* (Pocket Books, $1.75). They say it works.

Mild or occasional social drinking appears to be relatively harmless, and a wine nightcap might even be a safe soporific, but excessive alcohol consumption can be devastating to sleep.

According to a publication from the Sleep-Wake Disorders Unit at New York's Montefiore Hospital, "The sleep of alcoholics is characterized by many nighttime awakenings, low total sleep time, lower than normal amounts of Stage III or IV of Non-REM and of REM sleep, and a higher frequency of changes between states and stages of sleep."

In other words, alcohol makes sleep erratic. The irony is that many heavy drinkers originally took to the bottle in order to help a sleep problem. In so doing they gradually stepped up their intake to combat the body's growing tolerance, and eventually became habituated. Some doctors postulate that "alcoholism may permanently disturb the sleep mechanism."

As is the case with other drugs, sudden withdrawal from alcohol can be hazardous. A doctor or the local chapter of Alcoholics Anonymous should be consulted if the addiction to alcohol is serious. Heavy drinkers who wish to cut down but not abstain entirely, or to whom an occasional drink seems to be a professional or social necessity, may find help, without being labelled alcoholics, from an organization called Drinkwatchers, Inc. Founded by two AA dropouts, Drinkwatchers is said to be excellent for executives who find themselves in business situations where teetotalling is a handicap.

For information, write Drinkwatchers, P.O. Box 1062, Burlingame, California, 94010. Suggested reading: *How to be a Drinkwatcher,* by Aeriel Winters ($6.95 from Box 179, Haverstraw, NY 10927); or *How to Control Your Drinking,* by William Miller and Ricardo Munoz (Prentice-Hall, $8.95).

These specific medical problems are probably responsible for only a fraction of sleep difficulties. In the great majority of cases, it is impossible to pinpoint one specific physiological cause. In their search for universal factors that might be present in all cases of insomnia, researchers have been probing the biochemical and physiological parameters of sleep. So far, the most significant finding has been the isolation of the brain chemical serotonin, which is definitely involved with the onset of sleep. They speculate that insomniacs may have difficulty converting serotonin from its amino acid precursor, l-tryptophan. (See the section on l-tryptophan in chapter five.) Degeneration of brain cells has also been mentioned as a possible universal factor, but so far nothing conclusive has been discovered.

One general factor that probably causes, or contributes to the system's inability to shift in and out of sleep properly is stress. What that is, and how to deal with it, is covered in the next chapter.

While doctors who keep up with the latest research have begun using natural alternatives, the overwhelming majority of physicians still treat sleep problems by automatically dispensing sleeping pills. The fact that drugs for inducing sleep are dangerous is still not universally accepted. Consequently, many patients are seeking alternative healing procedures not just for insomnia, but for all manner of ailments. Of the drugless therapies that are gaining favor, several, including chiropractic and homeopathy, are reported to have helped people sleep better.

Chiropractic

Chiropractic is the largest drugless healing profession in the world. Most people, however, think of chiropractors as "bone doctors" or "back crackers." Chiropractors consider themselves nerve specialists. They often employ a wide range of natural treatments—nutrition, hydrotherapy, exercise, and so forth—but their special training is in adjusting the vertebrae of the spinal column.

According to chiropractic theory, misalignment of the vertebrae can interfere with the activity of the nervous system, since it is from the spinal column that nerves branch out to the brain and to all the organs and glands of the body. The spinal column is, so to speak, the central switchboard. Chiropractors believe that the nervous system regulates the body's natural healing powers. By removing impediments to its proper functioning, they feel, we can enable the body to cure, or at least hasten recovery from disease.

According to several insomniacs we interviewed, occasional chiropractic adjustments have helped their sleep. They reported feeling less tense for some period after an adjustment. Chiropractors might also help with any posture problem that might interfere with sleep, and they are often good sources of advice on nutrition.

Chiropractors have had an image of quackery about them. In fact, few of their procedures have been well documented. However, they seem to be well trained and competent at their specialty. Problems enter the picture when chiropractors and their patients lose sight of the limitations of the practice.

A recommendation by a physician is the best way to find a good chiropractor. Most states have chiropractic associations and licensing boards. You might want to obtain a recommendation from one. For additional information, contact the American Chiropractic Association; 2200 Grand Ave., Des Moines, Iowa, 50312, or the International Chiropractic Association; 741 Brady St.; Davenport, Iowa, 52808.

Homeopathy

Several insomniacs reported good, long-range results with homeopathy. Homeopathic procedures are much the same, in theory, as the use of vaccines—they stimulate symptoms so that the body can purge itself of illness. However, infinitesimal quantities of compounds are used, and those are derived from plant, animal, and mineral sources. Basic to the treatments are the principal elements found in the body: sodium, potassium, iron, calcium, magnesium, phosphorus, sulfur, iodine, and others.

Like chiropractic, homeopathy has its detractors in the medical community. It was, however, once a widely used and reputable field, and is now in the process of regaining some of its lost credibility. While little scientific research has been done on its procedures, homeopathy appears to be harmless—if a treatment doesn't work, it just doesn't work. But, proponents claim, it won't do any harm.

Homeopaths boast a wide range of remedies for different types of insomnia. If you wish to consult with one, you can obtain a list of the best-trained homeopaths from the American Institute of Homeopathy, 6231 Leesburg Pike, Falls Church, Virginia, 22044.

CHAPTER FIVE

STRESS AND SLEEP
How to relieve
stress and tension

The pace of modern life, with its accompanying pressures, rapid changes, air pollution, excessive noise, and other unnatural impingements that disturb the balance of our nervous systems, encourages a general disruption of the body. The overtaxed system is constantly trying to regain its equilibrium in the face of overstimulation and disturbing forces. The endocrine and nervous systems are particularly disrupted by stress. Reportedly, brain cells deteriorate under excessive strain.

Stress has been studied by a number of researchers. We know quite precisely how it affects our bodies, our minds, and, by extension, our sleep. The General Adaption Syndrome, first described by Dr. Hans Selye, the renowned expert on stress, goes like this: When a stressful situation occurs—an attack by a mugger, a reprimand from your boss, a traffic jam; or even something pleasant but overwhelming, like winning a lottery or walking into a room and having a hidden crowd yell "surprise!"—the adrenal and pituitary glands begin to secrete hormones that both protect the body from injury and muster up strength from stored sugars and fats. Energy is mobilized. Respiration and blood pressure soar, muscles tense, pupils dilate. These and other automatic responses were instilled in us by nature to prepare the threatened body for either "fight or flight."

Our ancestors had everyday stressors that required violent reactions—attacks by wild beasts, for example. In the modern world most stressors are not the sorts of things that one flees from or fights. Our highly mobilized bodies do not *use* the powerful resources that are summoned. If we reject a response too often, the result is more-or-less permanent damage. Destruction of tissues and organs and an overall weakening of the endocrine and nervous systems result. One definition of stress is simply, "the wear and tear caused by life."

In extreme cases, heart disease or hypertension, or any of a number of serious psychosomatic illnesses—maybe even cancer—result from stress directly. For most of us, however, general tension is the result. It is as though the body were in a state of perpetual mobilization.

Undoubtedly, the stress-induced imbalances in the system affect the sleep mechanism. The *Journal of Human Stress* (September 1976) reports two clinical studies in which stress factors were found to disturb sleep. One study showed a decrease in the percentage of Stage IV sleep, and the other showed measurable REM disturbance after the subjects were exposed to stressful situations. This should not be surprising. Stress creates an aroused, hypermetabolic state; sleep is an *un*aroused, *hypo*metabolic state.

In the last few years the search for ways in which to combat stress has become increasingly intense. Relaxation techniques, exercise, and unorthodox medical practices have all been explored. In the rest of this chapter we will discuss a variety of techniques and procedures that are widely advocated to alleviate the effects of stress and, as a result, have beneficial influences on sleep. We have selected those that are considered valuable, as well as those that have attracted serious attention.

Where possible we provide step-by-step instructions that you can follow on your own, immediately. In other cases where the services of trained experts are required, we provide enough information for you to understand the subject and to locate the appropriate experts.

Do not expect overnight miracles from these procedures. Most of them have generalized effects on the nervous system, and, for the most part, are not intended to remove isolated symptoms. There should be no bad side effects; we alert you where caution should be employed. See the reading list for more detailed information.

Relaxation Therapy

Tension is the twin of insomnia. Invariably, the person who suffers with sleep problems at night is subject to nervousness, worry, anxiety, and fear during the day. Eliminating tension from both the skeletal, or external muscles, and the visceral muscles—the muscles of the internal organs—is an important step in acquiring sound sleep.

Doctors have concluded that nearly every person has some neuromuscular tension, detectable by instruments even when he thinks he is completely relaxed. You have probably noticed that, even when lying perfectly still in bed, your muscles maintain a certain degree of rigidity. Prior to sleep, your muscles should be limp, not rigid.

A great number of techniques have been developed for relaxing those tense muscles. Most of them involve efforts of the mind, and many of those, we feel, border on the strenuous. Without proper supervision, some instructions given by well-meaning writers might result in persons straining their minds in an attempt to achieve relaxation. Steer clear of anything that might lead to strain, for that, obviously, will have the opposite effect from the one intended—it will make you tense. It could even create a breakdown in mind-body coordination.

Of the techniques that seem relatively innocent and potentially effective, many are best done in bed, to court sleep when it is desired. The same holds true for other tension-relievers, like massage, or certain foods and drinks, which we will discuss in later chapters.

Of all the relaxation techniques that have gained attention in recent years, the Progressive Relaxation method is the most widely used and highly regarded, with the possible exception of the Transcendental Meditation program, which we discuss separately.

Some 35 years ago, Dr. Edmund Jacobson of the Laboratory for Clinical Physiology developed a technique for removing the "residual tension" that we mentioned earlier. Progressive Relaxation involves learning to recognize the signs of muscular contraction and cultivating the ability to eliminate increasingly deeper levels of tension.

In *How to Sleep Well*, Dr. Samuel Gutwirth, a student of Dr. Jacobson's, writes:

> Insomnia is always accompanied by a sense of residual tension and can always be surmounted when one is successful in discontinuing contraction of the muscles even in this minute degree. Abolishing residual tension is, then, the essential feature in learning to relax scientifically.

Eight Steps Toward Relaxing for Sleep

• Once a day, set aside practice periods of 45 minutes to an hour, just before or just after a meal. Arrange not to be disturbed. Loosen your clothing. Lie down on a wide bed or couch in a quiet room (it need not be dark) with your arms at your side, palms down, several inches from your body. Do not fold your hands or cross your legs. Close your eyes gently and easily—do not try to shut them tightly.

• Now relax by letting your weight sink into the bed. Do not *try* to relax, do not try talking to yourself in order to facilitate settling down. Dr. Gutwirth makes a point of distinguishing this method from autosuggestion. After about ten minutes, slowly stiffen the muscles in both arms without moving your arms and without clenching your fists. The stiffening should be done slowly, without putting undo stress on the muscles. Hold at a slight degree of stiffness for about ten seconds. Now stiffen a little more and hold for another ten seconds. Again stiffen and hold, this time for about 30 seconds.

• Carefully observe how your arms feel. You should notice a dull, taut sensation. This is indicative of contracted muscles and active nerves. Becoming aware of this sensation—the signs of muscular tension—is the first step in relaxation therapy.

• Now allow your arms to relax slowly, a little at a time. Notice how the taut sensation begins to diminish in intensity. Enjoy this relaxed state for five minutes.

● Repeat the entire procedure—stiffening and holding in progressive stages, becoming aware of the sensations, and then slowly relaxing.

● Repeat a third time.

● After the third repetition continue to let your arms relax. Relax them further and further, past the point where they felt relaxed initially.

Relaxation therapy, it should be noted, is the opposite of an exercise or an activity during which the muscles are contracted. It is a procedure of doing less and less. The key is to *let* yourself relax, not to *make* yourself relax.

Once you have mastered the above procedures, do the same with other muscle groups—the legs, chest, abdomen, and facial muscles. Always tense them and relax them in the same systematic manner that you followed with your arms. After a while you should be able to achieve a deep state of muscular relaxation quickly. Then you should be able to discontinue the period of tensing that precedes the relaxation. That is done at first to acquaint you with the contrasting sensations of tension and relaxation. Eventually, you should be able to lie down and completely relax every muscle group without effort.

According to Dr. Jacobson, the muscles of the eyes and face are particularly important for those who have sleep difficulties. They are, customarily, among the last muscles groups to become relaxed. "When any person lies without sleeping," says Dr. Jacobson, "it is because he is using his eyes and his speech to imagine or to recall, to think, to solve problems or to engage in other forms of mental activity. I have found that if eyes and speech organs are really relaxed (as measured electronically) for even as short a time as 30 seconds, the person is asleep at the end of this time."

Here are two techniques for relaxing the eye and face muscles:

● Lie down as before and, with eyelids closed, wrinkle your forehead by *pulling up* your eyebrows. Hold this position for about a minute, familiarizing yourself with the feeling of tension in the forehead muscles. Then let the forehead relax gradually. Hold the muscles in this relaxed state for about five minutes. Now close your eyelids very tightly. Hold in that position for about 30 seconds, noting the tension in the eyelids. Then let your eyelids go. Relax for a few minutes. Do this repeatedly until you feel all the residual tension is gone. As with the other procedures, the initial period of tensing up should eventually be eliminated.

• Another technique for relaxing the eyes can be done at bedtime. Close your eyelids tightly, and, without moving your head, look up. Hold this position for about 30 seconds, observing the tension in your eye muscles and eyeballs. Now relax your eyes completely, letting them go limp in their sockets. Lie in this relaxed state for about five minutes. Repeat the entire process. Next, close your eyes tightly, as before, but this time look *down*. Again, do not move your head. Follow the usual procedure for noticing the sensations and then relaxing. Do the same by looking to the right and to the left, always with eyes tightly closed and the head stationary.

Dr. Jacobson said that some people could, under his procedures, learn to control sleep problems in a few weeks. Others might take months, he said, but after a year or so, sleep should continue to come easily to them. Once the method is mastered, the exercises described would no longer be necessary. All the steps of relaxation for all the muscle groups should then be triggered at once, putting the body in a condition that is receptive to sleep.

Dr. Gutwirth, too, reported great success with the methods described above. He claimed that insomniacs after a few weeks of practice find it easy to let go and relax when they go to bed.

We asked Dr. Peter Hauri of the Dartmouth sleep lab, for his professional opinion of the Jacobson method. He reports good results with some patients using PR. He offered this case history:

"A woman nearly nine months pregnant came to me visibly exhausted, unable to sleep for weeks. She had taken LeMaze training because she had always wanted a natural childbirth. The instructor told her that sleep and proper rest are crucial to a successful birth. From that moment on she could not sleep. When she came to me she was desperate. I taught her progressive relaxation and told her that it didn't make any difference if she slept or just lay there and rested. I emphasized that it's beneficial enough to just lie there quietly. Once she stopped trying and distracted herself with the progressive relaxation exercises, her insomnia vanished."

Dr. Hauri saw two values in progressive relaxation: One, it "actually does help a person to relax tense muscles. It is absolutely essential that a chronically tense person learn to relax. The longer some people stay in bed, the more tense they get. PR helps them eliminate that tension."

The second reason: "Actually, the majority of insomniacs are not chronically tense. The way in which PR helps these people is to keep their minds occupied with something else so that the body will naturally relax. The PR exercises will distract them enough so that they will not *try* to sleep, which is the worst thing an insomniac can do."

Dr. Hauri adds, however, that PR is "not always useful for my insomniac patients." He uses biofeedback, meditation, and "whatever technique the patient has least resistance to." In some cases, he said, his progressive relaxation people "try so hard to relax with the PR that they get exhausted." That kind of exhaustion does not lead to sleep.

It seems, overall, that the PR method is the most highly regarded of the techniques used for simple muscle relaxation. We believe that one of the reasons for this is the precise training sessions recommended for daytime use. If, in these sessions, the person can overcome the tendency to *try*, then there is less likelihood that straining will be employed, however subconsciously, at night. Try it, but remember: Let go, don't try to relax.

Meditation

Once thought of as mystical and obscure, or as counter-culture fads, meditation techniques from the East have since become better understood, and are now accepted as legitimate methods for alleviating stress and, in some cases, for bringing about significant personal growth. The acceptance of meditation has led some people to invent simulated versions of them, which have also attained some popularity.

We chose to describe the Transcendental Meditation program of Maharishi Mahesh Yogi for several reasons: we are familiar with it, having had our own sleep problems significantly aided by the practice; it is highly standardized, widely available, and easily learned by anyone; its effects go beyond muscular relaxation; no other meditation practice has received as high a level of credibility or acceptance from the scientific community.

The latter is of special importance. Scientific research has documented TM's effects on insomnia as well as many other problems. The claims being made for other practices have not been verified in laboratories. The only comparative studies that have been done have supported TM's claim that it is unique. Until all the evidence is in, we feel it advisable to go with a proven technique. TM is safe and effective.

Psychiatrist Harold Bloomfield, author of a best-selling book on TM, writes: "Middle-aged patients with complaints of chronic insomnia report improvement in their sleep patterns within the first two or three weeks of meditation. This improvement in their sleep tends to continue until night sedation is no longer necessary, even in previously severe insomnia."

Other doctors have reported that as a therapy for insomnia, the TM program is "simple to administer, immediately effective, stable over time, and without any unfavorable side effects."

There are dozens of testimonials about TM and insomnia, all of which sound like this one from Dr. Peter Salk, who said he was so tired during his medical school days that he felt chronically exhausted. "I couldn't go to bed because I couldn't let go of the day, but I was wasting time not being functional." After a few years of TM, he claims, he is "chronically rested" and requires much less sleep than he once did.

Dr. Bloomfield reports this case study, which he says is typical:

"A 23-year-old secretary had been suffering from insomnia for years. Having begun taking sleeping pills very regularly, she finally sought psychiatric help because she feared becoming addicted to the medicine. After three months of the TM program, she no longer required any medication. Now she falls asleep easily and sleeps soundly."

Psychologist Donald E. Miskiman, of the University of Alberta in Canada, studied a group of insomniacs who averaged 75.6 minutes before falling asleep. Thirty days after taking the TM course the average time of sleep onset dropped

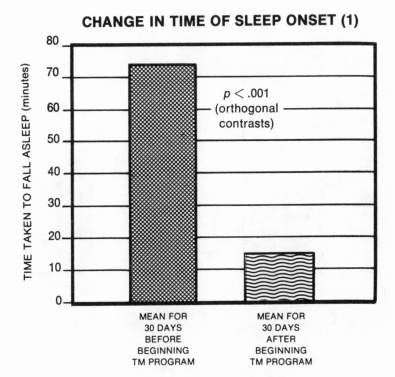

CHANGE IN TIME OF SLEEP ONSET (1)

to 15.1 minutes (see Figure 1).

Insomniacs who begin TM typically notice that they sleep for longer periods of time at first, as the body compensates for the previous loss of sleep. Within a week or two, normal sleep patterns tend to resume. Deeper sleep has been reported, as has the need for less total sleep time.

While improvement seems to come quickly, in many cases insomnia lingers. This might simply require patience and continued practice, or it might indicate that other procedures recommended in the book should also be employed. Don't expect overnight miracles from this or any other technique, and don't put all your eggs in one basket.

If the TM program does not substantially improve your sleep, it should at least help you cope with sleep loss. As illustrated in Figure 2, meditators who were subjected to 40 hours of sleep deprivation recovered more quickly than did a control group of nonmeditators, as measured by the amount of compensatory dreaming required once sleeping was resumed.

RESPONSE TO SLEEP DEPRIVATION (2)

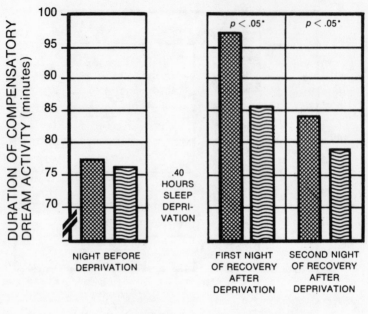

DURATION OF COMPENSATORY DREAM ACTIVITY (minutes)

100 — 95 — 90 — 85 — 80 — 75 — 70

.40 HOURS SLEEP DEPRIVATION

$p < .05$* $p < .05$*

NIGHT BEFORE DEPRIVATION

FIRST NIGHT OF RECOVERY AFTER DEPRIVATION

SECOND NIGHT OF RECOVERY AFTER DEPRIVATION

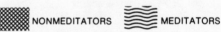

NONMEDITATORS   MEDITATORS

*ANALYSIS OF VARIANCE

Dr. Miskiman explained the phenomenon this way: "Transcendental Meditation seems to stabilize the sleep-dream cycle by reducing the effect of any disruption to this cycle and thereby restoring the system more quickly to its normal level of functioning."

TM, it should be noted, is not done before bed as a way to induce sleep. It is done for 20-minute periods, morning, and late afternoon to early evening, as a prelude to activity. Experience has shown that it will calm agitated persons enough to enable them to fall asleep, but that the energy boost it provides (it increases alertness) will come shortly, and the person will awaken refreshed. While this may be beneficial for daytime napping (and many insomniacs do nap during or after the practice) it is not advisable for the evening, as it will further disrupt the sleep/waking cycle. The technique's influence on nighttime sleep seems to be a carry-over from the two daytime sessions, and the permanent relief from stress.

Says biochemist, Dr. Carol Hart: "The person who meditates twice a day will relieve a lot of stress and strain. His body can then fall into a deep sleep at night without having to first relieve itself of those stresses."

Experiments on physiological changes such as oxygen consumption, heart rate, breath rate, skin resistance, lactate concentration, and other important variables, have verified that the TM technique produces an extraordinarily deep state of rest. (See Figure 3) This is said to enable the body to eliminate stress and strain that is so deeply rooted as to require extra deep rest for its removal. TM teachers say that this goes much deeper than relief from ordinary muscular tension, helping to "normalize" the brain and nervous system. Indeed, TM teachers, and most scientists well versed in the research, say that relaxation is only a minor aspect of TM's effects.

Studies show that the technique produces an unusually orderly, stable, and coherent style of brain functioning, as indicated by unprecedented brain-wave patterns. In addition, other studies report enhanced creativity, learning ability, reaction time, academic and job performance, and improve-

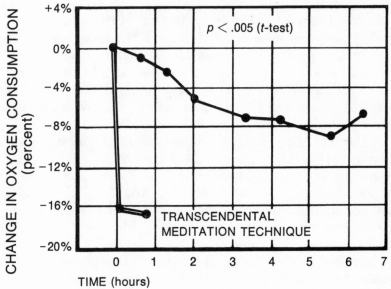

CHANGE IN METABOLIC RATE (3)

$p < .005$ (t-test)

TRANSCENDENTAL MEDITATION TECHNIQUE

CHANGE IN OXYGEN CONSUMPTION (percent)

TIME (hours)

ment on self-actualization measures. "Meditators make fewer mistakes, and suffer fewer frustrations," said one researcher, "which should make their heads more care free when they hit the pillow at night."

The TM technique is a mental one, requiring no changes in life-style, values or religious beliefs. Don't be put off by its Eastern origins, or in the private religious values of its founder, Maharishi Mahesh Yogi, a Hindu monk. It is quite compatable with Western ways, and is quite scientific in its approach.

TM is easy, and it requires no particular level of commitment or understanding; teachers refer to it as "automatic, natural, effortless." But, it must be learned through private instruction by a qualified teacher. No book can teach the technique properly, which is why we have not attempted to do so. The need for private instruction has been disputed by many who claim that the same basic results can be obtained through relaxation techniques that can be transmitted in writing. This, however, has not been proven. So far, research leans in TM's favor.

From our experience with people who have tried techniques taught in books, we have concluded that the simulated versions tend to be haphazard, incomplete at best, and often dangerous, for they leave the reader unguided. You can't ask a book a question. Moreover, there is too much room for misinterpretation. And, since meditation is a delicate instrument, anything can happen. One of the advantages of the TM program, aside from its scientific endorsement, is that it is taught by a large organization that provides precise instruction and ongoing guidance to the meditators. All in all, you are well advised to invest the time and money in the standard TM course rather than play around with an imitation.

The technique itself revolves around the mental use of sounds (without meaning) called *mantras*. The vibratory frequencies of these sounds, which have been handed down through an ancient and honorable tradition, are said to resonate harmoniously with the meditator's nervous system, bringing about the state of orderly, alert rest described earlier.

During private instruction, the TM teacher assigns a mantra individually, according to certain criteria which he will not divulge. The teacher then guides the student in proper use of the mantra through a series of steps, each of which depends on the student's experiences. Some have suggested that the mantras are arbitrary, and that any pleasant sound would suffice. TM teachers firmly insist that the selection of the mantra and the instructions for its use are matters of precision requiring training. A study at the Institute of Living in Hartford, Connecticut, found that the TM mantras produce different brain-wave effects than arbitrarily chosen sounds.

Free introductory presentations are offered to the public regularly by TM organizations affiliated under the World Plan Executive Council. After attending two lectures, you are eligible to take the actual TM course. The course requires only two hours a day for four consecutive days—one day for personal instruction, and three more of seminars. After that, the technique is yours to use, and extensive follow-up is available as needed. At this writing, the cost of the TM course—including the basic follow-up services—is $165. Standard discounts are available for students and families.

There are over 300 TM centers in the United States staffed by qualified instructors. Consult the Appendix for a list of major centers. Your telephone directory should list your local center under Transcendental Meditation, or International Meditation Society.

Biofeedback

Touted by its proponents as a spectacular breakthrough in science, biofeedback training has captured the attention of researchers throughout the world. Many see it as a sort of technological panacea with which we will eventually regulate our glandular secretions, control cancer, even remove warts—all through mind control.

In biofeedback, a person is hooked up to equipment that can monitor events in the body—brain waves, heartbeat, blood pressure, temperature, muscular tension, stomach acidity, and others. These events are translated into readily observable signals such as lights, tones, or wavy lines. Once a person can, as it were, "see" his heartbeats, or "hear" his brain activity, he has information that can, presumably, help him control those specific functions.

Dr. Peter Hauri outlines five basic steps involved in all biofeedback procedures:

"1) Measure a physiological parameter in a motivated subject.

2) Display (feed back) the measurement to the subject.

3) Usually by trial and error the subject learns (consciously or unconsciously) what behaviors change the display.

4) The subject is reinforced for changes in the correct direction, usually simply by seeing success.

5) With success, the subject learns (consciously or unconsciously) what internal cues are associated with the reinforced changes. He then no longer needs the feedback display, but can control the physiological parameter directly."

Biofeedback advocates claim that it can remedy certain ailments such as migraine headaches, tension, epilepsy, cardiac arrhythmias, and high blood pressure. Some practitioners say they have had dramatic success in treating insomnia. Dr. Thomas Budzynski of the University of Colorado, for example, has devised a training session in which insomniacs are taught to reproduce body-wave and brain-wave patterns associated with the onset of sleep. "With this training," Budzynski reports, "people who had taken four hours to fall asleep were dropping into slumber twice in a 20-minute lab session." He concludes, "I think doctors are going to lend patients an EMG machine instead of handing out sleeping pills in the future."

Despite such enthusiastic reports, however, judgment should be reserved. Dr. Hauri at Dartmouth, Dr. Sterman at U.C.L.A., Dr. Salamy at the University of Texas, and others, are doing work on biofeedback and sleep. Many claim to have had promising results, but it is too soon to judge biofeedback—all the evidence is not yet in, and serious doubts have been raised. Says Dr. Hauri, "Therapeutic claims often overstate beyond belief the small kernels of sound, scientific evidence found in laboratories and clinical research. Clinicians will do well to keep a keen, but very critical eye on future developments, guarding both against excessive gullibility and against wholesale rejection of the field (where excellent scientific work currently mingles with obvious quackery)."

The most reliable equipment for monitoring and reporting bodily signals is very expensive, cumbersome, and must be operated by skilled technicians. Less expensive machines promoted by commercial firms are often inaccurate and have led to serious, often dangerous reactions. Good machines also require constant, skilled adjustment.

Besides the machines themselves, doubts have been raised about the entire process. Dr. Solomon Steiner of the City University of New York points out that a wide variety of facial expressions such as blinking, twitching, raising of eyeballs, frowning, and gritting of teeth, can produce signals on brain-wave machines that are also associated with more important phenomena. Conceivably, a person who thinks he is training himself to control an important physical system, might end up a skilled twitcher, or worse.

Another objection to biofeedback is that trainees are often unable to sustain results in their daily lives away from the laboratory and the machines. Writes physiologist-physician, Charles Stroebel of a study comparing biofeedback to the Transcendental Meditation technique, "The alpha subjects (biofeedback trainees) experienced ... difficulty in transferring their training to environments outside the laboratory."

It is possible that being trained to induce sleep in a controlled setting will not help you fall asleep in your own bed. Also, it is conceivable that producing brain waves that happen to occur during sleep onset may not produce the same entire state as natural sleep. Sleep is, after all, a complex phenomenon, not just a particular set of brain waves. Biofeedback can only work on one variable at a time. Suppose you could deliberately produce the same brain waves that occur during, say, digestion, would it be the same as eating?

Skepticism also extends to questions about the possible side effects of artificially manipulating mind-body coordination in that manner, and about the use of elaborate equipment to do something that might be done more naturally and less expensively. Our fascination with machines and elaborate technology often blinds us to the fact that nature works in simple, elegant ways.

With these pros and cons in mind, you should be able to decide whether or not to look into biofeedback. The general consensus seems to be that it is a promising field, but that its main results so far have been in areas like muscle relaxation, where other, more accessible, methods seem superior. It is important to have some knowledge of biofeedback, because many doctors are quick to recommend it. If you are inclined to experiment with it, be sure to obtain your training from a reputable hospital or university, where you will be guided by trained medical personnel.

Exercise Your Way to Sleep

Mental and spiritual fitness, both dependent on a good brain, are greatly enhanced by optimal physical fitness. Body, mind, and soul are inextricably woven together, and whatever helps or hurts any one of these three sides of the whole man helps or hurts the other two.

—eminent cardiologist,
Paul Dudley White

When Theodore Dreiser was a struggling young writer suffering from insomnia, he got a job as a section hand on the New York Central Railway. After a day of driving spikes and shovelling gravel, he was so exhausted he could hardly stay awake long enough to eat dinner.

You needn't become a manual laborer in order to feel tired at bedtime. But, if you lead a sedentary sort of life during the day, it is a good bet that exercise will prove a significant aid in attaining better sleep. "Regular exercise promotes deep sleep," writes sleep researcher Quentin R. Regestein. "Insomniac patients should exercise vigorously and frequently." Research has established that vigorous exercise during the day, or mild exercise at bedtime, increases the amount of Stage IV sleep, the deepest part of the non-REM cycle.

Just about every insomniac to whom we suggested increased exercise claimed to have slept better when he followed the advice. One man claimed to have overcome the problem entirely. According to his story, his insomnia began at the time of an athletic injury in college, three years ago. The injury ended a promising basketball career, and threw the victim into a state of depression, to which he attributed his insomnia.

But the depression had long ago disappeared, the young man having adjusted to the life of an ex-athlete. Yet the sleeplessness continued. When he began exercising, more to lose some accumulated poundage than to improve his sleep, he noticed an improvement in his sleep immediately. He concluded that his body, accustomed to strenuous work all its life, sorely missed the daily workouts that ended with his injury.

Your body was meant to be used. If you don't move enough, your circulation and your breathing can become sluggish. Lactic acid, which is known to correlate with stress, accumulates in the blood. Tension builds in the muscles. The brain can even become dull.

Exercise is not only fun, but it charges the nervous system with vitality, activates the all-important endocrine glands, stimulates and strengthens internal organs such as the heart and lungs, and improves mental functioning. In addition, exercise seems to help lift the clouds of boredom, worry, and tension that contribute to sleep problems. In *Positive Addiction*, Dr. William Glasser states that the hormone epinephrine, a chemical that has been linked with feelings of happiness, doubles in the body after ten minutes of sustained exercise. This can result in long-lasting pleasurable effects.

More and more doctors are recommending vigorous exercise for their patients regardless of age, especially in cases where the patient does not move around much in the course of his regular routine. Here are some effective exercise programs, chosen on the basis of popularity, convenience, and effectiveness.

Jogging: This has become the most popular form of everyday exercise in the United States. Doctors have found that only 15 or 20 minutes of jogging four times a week will go a long way toward turning most people into good physical specimens. Specific ailments have been relieved by jogging. A well-known psychiatrist, Dr. Thaddeus L. Kostrubula, himself a faithful jogger, found that running triggered dramatic personality changes in some of his most difficult patients, including schizophrenics, chronic depressives, drug-abusers, and insomniacs. He also found that the more people jog, the more vividly they dream, and the more their deeper emotions become accessible to their conscious awareness. Those findings have been verified by others, and should be encouraging to any insomniacs—chronic or occasional—who suspect that emotional factors may be contributing to their problem.

Jogging is a form of "aerobic" exercise, a term made popular by Dr. Kenneth Cooper, whose books on aerobics have sold nearly two million copies. The word means, literally, "with oxygen." Aerobic exercises consist of constant, strenuous movement that builds up the body's capacity for utilizing oxygen. Among other things, the efficient use of oxygen is essential for a well-functioning liver, the impairment of which many feel contributes to insomnia.

Aerobics—including swimming, bicycling, and brisk walking—are best known for their strengthening effect on the heart and lungs. Dr. Cooper relates many case histories and scientific experiments that support the contention that regular aerobic exercise will help almost anyone overcome maladies as serious as heart disease and as insidious as insomnia. They are being used increasingly by busy executives, in whose companies well-equipped gymnasiums are becoming a common sight.

If you are not used to regular exercise, don't start by entering the Boston Marathon. Start gradually. Dr. Willibald Nagler of Cornell's College of Medicine warns that too much jogging too soon can be dangerous. "It takes at least six months for a sedentary man to become a good jogger," he writes. "Don't make any sudden changes in your exercise routine."

If you are over 30, get a check-up before you begin a regular jogging program. If you have heart problems, or are over 50, have your doctor administer an electrocardiogram (EKG) to test your endurance. Many doctors recommend having a stress test, which involves running on a treadmill or pedalling on a stationary bike while your heart rate, EKG, blood pressure, and oxygen consumption are measured.

Begin with some light calisthenics (jumping jacks are good) and easy stretching motions. Then set off at an easy shuffle. Jog at a comfortable pace for as long as you feel you are not straining. Dr. Nagler recommends five to ten minutes a day to start with. If your breathing becomes labored, or if you feel any pain, slow down to a walk. Keep walking briskly until you feel recovered, then jog again. For the first week or so, it would probably be wise to limit your session to ten or 15 minutes, giving yourself plenty of time to wind down slowly. Always end your jogging with a period of leisurely walking around, to allow the blood in your legs a chance to circulate to the rest of your body. Never sit down immediately after jogging. If, after running, you feel dizzy or have pains, discontinue and see your doctor. If you note that you feel stimulated after exercise, avoid exercising close to bedtime.

While jogging does relax the muscles, late evening jogging may speed up your body just when you want it to slow down. A good time to jog is early in the morning before breakfast (never exercise after a meal), when the air is its freshest and cleanest. Many doctors recommend late afternoon to early evening as especially refreshing after a hard day behind a desk. Some studies have shown that vigorous exercise at that time can increase the percentage of Stages III and IV of sleep.

If you find jogging boring, or if you have problems finding the discipline to jog, you might like to run with a partner or a group. If so, and if you have only lazy acquaintances, contact the National Jogging Association; P.O. Box 19367; Washington, D.C. 20036. They will let you know of jogging groups in your vicinity.

Nice alternatives for those who are pressed for time, or for when the weather is foul, are the Home Jogger and the Pacer-Mat Physical Modulator Mini-trampoline, or trampolettes. These playthings make for great exercise and lots of fun. They help you avoid the wear and tear of jogging on hard surfaces, and can double as focal points for sheer enjoyment. We have seen men and women of all shapes, sizes, and physical conditions gleefully bouncing around their dens or living rooms. They say they get all the benefits of jogging too.

The Home Jogger is manufactured by Skip Helen Enterprises, 11259 Virginia Ave., Lynwood, California, 90262. The Pacer-Mat is manufactured by Tri-flex, 1208 Missouri Ave., S. Houston, Texas, 77587.

If the thought of running around in a sweatsuit in broad daylight is abhorrent to you, and if the Home Jogger is unappealing, here is an alternative.

Skipping rope: Not only little girls, but boxers and other athletes do it. Ropejumping is a remarkably complete, exhilarating exercise that helps build up lungs, heart, legs, arms and chest.

One of the advantages of this playful exercise, of course, is that it can be done indoors at any time, depending on who lives beneath you. Buy yourself a professional skip rope with ball bearings in the handles. It should be long enough to reach from armpit to armpit while passing under both feet. Skip on a soft surface such as a rug or mat, or wear shoes with a thick rubber sole. If you are out of shape, follow this advice from Dr. Lenore R. Zohman:

"[Step] over the rope one foot at a time, rather than bouncing over it with both feet. It's easier, and will prevent rapid increases in heart rate. It avoids ankle and foot discomfort too, which is common in new jumpers who are not conditioned to landing on both feet. The step-over method is very similar to the foot motions used in jogging."

Start with some light warmup exercise—stretching, doing jumping jacks, or jogging slowly in place. When you skip, learn how to come down on the balls of your feet in a "soft" landing. Relax so that your ankles, knees and hips are slightly bent. Wear loose-fitting clothes. And enjoy it—you might even skip to your favorite music, so long as it is not too fast a tempo. Be sure to cool down after a workout by walking around.

As with jogging, it is a good idea not to skip rope just before bedtime or after a large meal.

Walking: Perhaps the cheapest, easiest, and most accessible form of exercise is plain old walking. It just might be the best too.

Get into the habit of walking instead of relying on conveniences that save time but do little good for your body. Says Dr. Frederick J. Stare of Harvard, "The sedentary businessman should make exercise a part of his daily life. He ought to get into the habit, for instance, of walking instead of taking cabs for short rides. He ought to walk up a flight or two of stairs at the office instead of always taking the elevator." A brisk 15-or 20-minute walk in the open air brings nearly every muscle into play. Dr. Paul Dudley White, a dedicated walker, suggested walking at a pace of three to four miles per hour for a total of six or seven hours a week.

Dr. White emphasized the "importance of the use of the leg muscles as an integral part of the maintenance of a proper circulation." He claimed that studies have shown "that when a person is walking, about 30 percent of the circulation of the blood is carried on by the leg muscles, and the remaining percent by the heart." Vigorous use of the leg muscles also helps keep the veins free of clots.

Leg circulation has been found to have an important influence on sleep. Dr. White, speaking of using the leg muscles, said: "The fatigue produced by it is undoubtedly the best tranquilizer ever made, either by nature or man."

Insomniacs can verify this fact. The next time you have difficulty falling asleep, or when you awaken in the night, notice the feeling in your legs. Often, you will feel a sort of dull sensation, or a restlessness as though your legs want to move, even though the rest of you wants to sleep. You might have the urge to massage your legs. If any of these signs are present, it is a good bet that leg circulation is playing a role in keeping you awake. Massage, or stretching, or walking around the room will help at the time. But regular exercise is essential.

When you go out walking, walk with a loose-jointed roll. Swing your arms freely and swing easily from one foot to the other with a skatinglike motion. Walk briskly and walk often.

Other exercises: There are a great many forms of exercise, of course. Those we described are easy and popular, and have been found to be of definite benefit to sleep. The important thing is that you take *some* form of regular exercise, preferably aerobic, to keep your body functioning smoothly and to help bring about normal fatigue at night.

Swimming is excellent. Most areas have Y's and health clubs with good-sized pools. Some people prefer competitive sports like squash or tennis. The trouble there is that it requires a partner, and one is not always available. You might persuade a friend to make a regular committment. If you depend on golf, by the way, it will serve the purpose only if you walk between holes.

An excellent, carefully structured exercise program, ideal for the busy person since it requires only ten or 11 minutes a day, is the Royal Canadian Air Force Program. The exercises are carefully graded and can be done at home or in the office. Pick up a copy of *Royal Canadian Air Force Exercise Plans for Physical Fitness* (Pocket Books, $1.75). Follow the instructions to the letter. They are proven.

Fitness Publications has a book called *Fitness Management*, written by Vincent W. Antonelli, a business executive and lecturer on fitness. It has good exercise advice, and a quantitative program that takes weight loss, age, sex, body build, and physical condition into account. Write to P.O. Box 1786, Poughkeepsie, N.Y. 12601. It costs $4.50.

However you decide to do it, get at least some exercise during the day. You should notice the difference in bed.

Daytime Naps for Nighttime Sleep

The eccentric genius, Salvador Dali, sits in a chair holding a spoon loosely between his fingers. On the floor beneath the dangling spoon he places a tin plate. He closes his eyes. Sleep comes, the spoon falls, and the clatter of metal jolts the artist into wakefulness. Dali claims that he is completely refreshed by the sleep he gets from the time the spoon leaves his hand until it hits the plate.

Less bizarre, but unusual nonetheless, was Eleanor Roosevelt's habit of stealing a furtive one-minute snooze while sitting perfectly upright at a dinner party. She was also said to nap regularly on speaker's platforms, always awakening just before she was introduced.

It might take some time and luck before you gain the napping proficiency of Dali or Mrs. Roosevelt, but acquiring the skill might do more for your insomnia than a bookful of medical advice; it will help alleviate the aftermath of a fitful night, and may also help prevent further trouble the next night.

The question of napping for insomniacs is a disputed point. Some experts recommend it, while others are unequivocally opposed to it and consider napping detrimental to evening slumber. When we visited the sleep clinic at Montefiore Hospital, Dr. Pollack, our attending physician, told us to give up afternoon naps. When we objected, he explained that he wanted to change our rather erratic bed-time schedules, which varied as much as three hours from one night to the next. He wanted to establish a regular rhythm, which is apparently important for chronic insomniacs. He offered the choice of eliminating naps or instituting them as a daily routine at the same time every day.

From all indications, napping is an individual matter, good for some insomniacs, not good for others. If you have initial insomnia (difficulty falling asleep), and are accustomed to a regular nap, you might do well to eliminate it for at least long enough to see if it is, in fact, interfering with your sleep. During this experiment, go to bed at the same time every night.

Napping might be especially good if yours is the type of insomnia that awakens you prematurely and unrefreshed. Your internal rhythms may be better suited to early rising with a compensatory 40 winks during the day than to the standard eight solid hours at night. One insomniac we know, who had tried a number of remedies to no avail, finally found that a good nap after lunch was all he needed.

"I used to get up at dawn unable to fall back to sleep," he said. "I was okay for a few hours but then I would be overcome by fatigue and drag through the rest of the day. Often I would collapse in bed, exhausted, but unable to sleep through the whole night. Finally, in desperation, I cut my lunch hour short and added a nap. If I oversleep, my boss lets me make up the time later on. I work more effectively now, and I don't mind waking up at dawn. In fact, I sort of like it."

The widespread belief that an afternoon nap will make you too alert to fall asleep at night is not true for everyone. Overexhaustion can actually hinder natural sleep. Dr. Philip Tiller of the Louisiana State School of Medicine induced several hundred women who had complained of being nervous, fatigued, and generally run down, into taking a one- or two-hour nap every afternoon. He determined experimentally that the naps helped the women sleep better at night. About two-thirds of the women reported a significant decrease in other symptoms as well.

Some believe that naps shorter than two hours are not restful since the body does not have time to go through the entire non-REM and REM cycle. This has been disputed.

"You don't need certain amounts of REM or slow-wave [Stage IV] sleep to function effectively," stated one scientist. "This idea prevailed until the late 1950s and '60s. But it has been disproven."

Like a small diamond, even a small nap can be of tremendous value. Writes psychologist Ray Giles in, *Our Human Body:* "Fifteen minutes of sleep after the heaviest work and before the main meal count more for efficiency than five times as much late, light sleeping in the morning."

Don't feel guilty if you decide to tune out for a few minutes in the middle of the day. You will be in good company. Most cultures have institutionalized rest periods of greater length than our own lunch and coffee breaks. They are much more tranquil too. According to the *New York Times*, it is not uncommon in China to find shops closed, workers away from their jobs, and people sleeping along the streets and alleyways anytime between 11:00 AM and 3:00 PM.

History's artful nappers include such great achievers as Thomas Edison, who slept for five hours and catnapped as needed, General Douglas MacArthur, Napoleon, Winston Churchill, and modern presidents Truman, Eisenhower, Kennedy, and Johnson. Wrote Churchill in *The Gathering Storm:*

> I always went to bed at least for one hour as early as possible in the afternoon and exploited to the full my happy gift of falling almost immediately to sleep. By this means I was able to press a day and a half's work into one. Nature had not intended mankind to work from eight in the morning until midnight without the refreshment of blessed oblivion, which, even if it lasts only 20 minutes, is sufficient to renew all vital forces.

Among the more contemporary nappers are former Secretary of State, Henry Kissinger, who is known to be able to fall asleep sitting upright in a plane, and Barbara Walters, who says that she can fall asleep in any chair, or in a plane or train. "If I sleep for more than an hour, I wake feeling tired," says the news personality, "But it's always better for me to get some sleep than none at all."

One reason that napping can improve normal sleep at

night is that it can help your day go better, thus leaving you with fewer cares. Dr. Charles Fisher, a New York psychoanalyst who has been researching sleep for some 25 years, writes: "We still don't know, scientifically, why so short a sleep—ten minutes, one minute—can be refreshing to many people. Obviously, it relaxes the muscles. But what else? It could be that it stops conscious thought processes, and in this way relieves anxiety. Or, as has been found, nondreaming sleep helps the problem-solving mechanism."

Another explanation has to do with oscillating tension levels. "Tension increases as the day goes on," reports William Kitay, in *The Challenge of Medicine*. "If the business executive breaks it at noon with a short nap the tension curve drops to near base line, and he awakens for the work of the afternoon refreshed."

How to Sleep on the Job

Many executives are doing just that, whether they are at the office or not. "I've trained myself to go to sleep instantly so I can get a few minutes' rest while riding in a plane or car," says Harding Lawrence, Chairman of the Board of Braniff International Airlines. "Just that refreshes me a great deal."

Not every boss will be amenable to your taking naps, of course. Charles J. Pilliod, Chairman of the Board of Goodyear, while admitting that he could "grab 40 winks under almost any circumstances and feel refreshed," would not like any one of his employees to follow suit. Said Mr. Pilliod of napping on company time, "I would figure he needed the rest of the afternoon off, probably the next morning, and maybe a long time after that."

A little logic, and a sincere attitude, might be all you need to convince your boss of the advantages of letting you nap during office hours. Many companies, in fact, have infirmaries with cots which employees are welcome to use if they feel the need for a snooze.

The best time to nap is said to be just after lunch, the traditional siesta time. If that is impossible, any time in the afternoon will do. According to German psychiatrist-neurologist, Uros Jovanovic, "People need to take a nap some time between 1:00 P.M. and 3:00 P.M. to maintain full efficiency." If you decide to experiment with napping, settle on a convenient time and take your nap every day at that same time. Regularity is important.

You needn't have a proper bedroom to nap in, although that might be preferable. A sofa, the carpeted floor in your office, or even a comfortable chair will serve the purpose. Some people keep a fold-away cot or a foam rubber pad in their offices, along with a blanket and pillow.

Having conjured up a comfortable situation, draw the shades, take the phone off the hook, put a *Do Not Disturb* sign on your door. Lie down, close your eyes, and put aside your pressing thoughts for a moment. You needn't worry about losing them. If they are really important, they will be there when you wake up and you will be better able to deal with them. Take a few deep breaths, relax, and lie there until sleep comes.

How long should your nap be? Dr. Jovanovic says that "an afternoon nap should not be less than 20 minutes long nor more than 90 minutes." Let your body indicate for itself what length is best for you.

If you've set a napping schedule, try to find time to lie down at the predetermined hour every day, even if you do not feel sleepy at the time. Give yourself at least 15 minutes. Even if you don't fall asleep, just lying there will be remarkably refreshing.

Your Job and Your Sleep

Most of us spend about one-third of our lives at work. Our experiences there—our successes and failures, our satisfactions and frustrations, our working conditions, our relationships with our fellow workers—all these, and more, have a significant effect on our sleep. So much stress is incurred on the job that corporations by the dozen are investigating ways to cut down stress factors for their employees. Here are some things to keep in mind about relating that vital eight hours of your life to sleep.

Two categories of workers have virtually chronic sleep disorders but accept them as "normal" for people in their occupations: shift workers, and those who cross time zones regularly.

Studies have shown that when you take normal, healthy subjects and reverse their sleep-wake cycles, they begin to have frequent awakenings and can't sustain normal sleep. People who work at night and sleep during the day often suffer severe sleep difficulties that require only a change in schedule to fix. Nature may not have intended for them to be owls.

Moreover, night-shifters often have their problems compounded because their families and friends do not work at night. Thus, their homes are noisy and active when they are trying to sleep. Perhaps more important, they feel deprived of normal family and social pleasures, and further disturb their sleep by trying to remain awake, say, when their children come home from school. Typically, they try to revert to sleeping at night with everyone else on weekends and holidays. This only further compounds the poor adaptation of their bodies.

Most severely affected are those workers who are called upon to change shifts often. Many industries have their employees rotate day and night shifts. Doctors, nurses, policemen, firemen—all are typically called upon to be awake when their bodies think it is time to sleep.

The solution? It's a trade-off. Individuals and companies, and society at large must come to terms with priorities. Perhaps, in nonessential areas, it might be worth a small slowdown of production for the sake of complying with nature's intentions.

Pilots, flight attendants, and everyone else involved in jet travel, as well as businessmen, athletes, and others who jet around regularly, have to deal with jet-lag. As a result of crossing time zones, their usual sleep-wake rhythms are often out of sync with their localities. The businessman who flies from San Francisco to New York, for example, might find himself unable to get to sleep because it is only 8:00 in his body even though it is 11:00 on his hotel clock. It might take days or weeks to readjust. Unfortunately, before that happens the person is likely to be long gone to another time zone, only to have the same problem there.

The solution? More intelligent scheduling, taking into account the available data and your own individual experience in adjusting to jet-lag. According to some critics, airlines have been cavalier about their employee's flight schedules, paying more attention to costs than health. The same might be true in other industries where constant travel is required.

One proposed solution is to have the traveler maintain his or her clock in tune with a single time zone. That is, not to try to adapt to each new location, but to continue to sleep according to the time of his most frequent location, preferably that of his home. While this may hamper a person's social life while travelling, and while it may make business meetings more difficult to schedule to everyone's convenience, it might be well worth it. Allegedly, Soviet air crews on the Moscow-to-Havana run stay sequestered in a compound when they are in Havana; the compound is always on Moscow time.

Most shift-workers and constant travelers are aware of the cause of their sleeplessness. It is perfectly obvious to them. However, they frequently try to overcome it with sleeping pills. Suppose that San Francisco businessman, for example, is lying awake at midnight thinking about a 9:00 A.M. meeting. He gets anxious about being tired at that time, and pops a pill thinking he will get to sleep faster.

The night-worker who wants to be able to get to sleep at the same time as his family on Saturday night so he can spend Sunday with them, also may resort to pills. In either case, the pill may, indeed, put the person to sleep, but he is not likely to feel at his best in the morning.

Fitting Work Hours to Sleep Needs

Try to arrange your working hours to fit your sleep needs. This is not always easy to do, of course, if your sleep needs keep you too far removed from the 9:00 to 5:00 day that most people expect of you. But, depending on your position, you will be surprised at how easy it might be to rearrange your schedule. Bill Forman is a salesman for a large manufacturing company. Every morning he would awaken at about 4:00, perfectly refreshed. However, he needed a good, solid nap in the afternoon. If he did not get it, he would be foggy and dull. Unfortunately, he did not feel right taking a nap during working hours, and so he just trudged through as best he could. Finally, it got unbearable, and his boss was not pleased about his performance—Mr. Forman excelled at some things, and was dismal at others.

Forman and the boss had a long talk, the upshot of which was that the salesman scheduled all his meetings with customers for the period between 9:00 A.M. and 1:00 P.M. and was allowed to do all his paperwork whenever convenient. For Mr. Forman, that meant he could do his paperwork very early in the morning and nap in the afternoon. Boss and salesman were both delighted.

Try not to rely on an alarm clock. Waking prematurely to that harsh sound, day in and day out, can wreck your system, for it will be interrupting important functions of sleep. Remember what we said earlier about REM deprivation. You might try getting to sleep earlier and waking naturally. Or arrange for more flexible morning hours of work.

It is very important to end your work day well in advance of bedtime. You should ease into sleep, not crash into it. Many busy executives have difficulty getting to bed at night, for the simple reason that they work right until they brush their teeth. A corporate vice president named Jack Bunker, even listened to tapes of business conferences while washing up at bedtime. Then he would read reports in bed. Needless to say, it took him so long to fall asleep that he kept a vial of sleeping pills handy on his end table. It was only the onset of ulcers that got him to reevaluate his habits. The first thing his doctor told him was to leave all his work at the office. Within a few weeks, he was sleeping relatively easily and did not refill his sleeping pill prescription.

So, fill the pre-bed hours with something pleasant, soothing, and unstrained. Take your spouse to bed with you, not your work.

Pacing yourself properly is also important. Your job should have breaks built into it, and decent vacation opportunities. Don't overdo it. Many an ambitious person has driven himself to success only to discover that he is too tired, or too sick, to enjoy it. Set your goals realistically. Evaluate yourself and your situation and set goals that are ambitious, but within reasonable grasp. Work hard, but work sensibly. "I have never known a person who suffered from overwork," states Dr. Joseph F. Montague, "I have, however, treated many patients who have suffered from overtrying—from having too big an ambition, an exaggerated goal."

A hard day's work can either make you sleep like a babe or keep you tossing and turning all night. According to Dr. Hans Selye, the renowned expert on stress, "A stressful activity which has come to a definite stop prepares you for rest and sleep; but one which sets up self-maintaining tensions keeps you awake."

Dr. Selye offers this vocational advice for insomniacs:

"Do not let yourself get carried away and keyed up more than is necessary to acquire the momentum for the best performance of what you want to do in the interest of self-expression.

"Keep in mind that the hormones produced during acute stress are meant to alarm you and key you up for peak accomplishments. They tend to combat sleep.

"Try not to overwork any one part of your body or mind disproportionately by repeating the same actions to exhaustion. Be especially careful to avoid the senseless repetition of the same task when you are already exhausted."

It is important not to strive for accomplishments that you are not ready to attain comfortably. To an ambitious person, there is a delicate line to tread—it lies between working to one's capacity and straining beyond it. The former is exhilarating, the latter is devastating. Says Professor Eugene E. Jennings of the Michigan State School of Business Administration, "A man who is working ahead of his capabilities is living on a razor's edge. It's the hairiest kind of life there is."

Know your limits, then, and know what you are ready for. Set your sights high, but be realistic about your timetable for getting there, always remembering that if you lose too much sleep on the way you'll be too exhausted to enjoy yourself when you arrive.

Your work should also be enjoyable. Far too many people spend eight hours a day wishing they were somewhere else. They seethe inside, the tension builds, and they end up spending half their nights fantasizing about fabulous jobs and exotic places, or mentally telling off everyone, from their boss to their clients and colleagues. It is not asking too much of life to work at a job that you like, especially if not doing so prevents you from obtaining one of nature's pleasures—a good night's sleep. Career change is quite acceptable nowadays, and the bookshelves are filled with good advice on how to go about it. We recommend *What Color is Your Parachute?* by Boles.

Experts are distinguishing between *dys*stress and *eu*stress. Dystress consists of the noxious pressures of work, the kind that are dangerous and can lead to serious illness or emotional disturbance. Eustress (eu is in "euphoria") refers to those stimuli that are interesting, challenging, and necessary for self-expression. These are the kind that persons of accomplishment thrive on, and without which life would be dull.

Many corporations are actively trying to minimize dystress and maximize eustress. You should do the same with your life. It is an important distinction to remember, because so many people, in trying to eliminate stress from their lives, end up eliminating all challenges. They dream of being on a desert island with absolutely nothing to do. They don't realize that boredom and monotony can be stressful—ruts are a major source of insomnia. The mysterious "weekend insomniacs," who only have sleep problems when they are not working, are quite likely bored. They lack an outlet for their energies, which, going unreleased, keep them wired up at night.

Keep happily busy, therefore, with challenging, constructive work, and with hobbies and social activities that you enjoy. The latter is important. Boston housewife, Mary Platt was always a sound sleeper until her three children were grown and gone away from home. Then she suddenly developed insomnia. It was more than the customary change in sleep patterns that comes with age, the doctors agreed. After the usual factors were eliminated, they finally suspected that Mrs. Platt was simply bored and feeling useless. They pushed her into active pursuit of interesting activities. She was a particularly giving type of person, so she found civic organizations a decent replacement for the chores of a mother. She also got a boost out of taking piano lessons again. She got so busy, in fact, that her sleep was threatened by overwork. When she struck a happy medium, her sleep was restored to normal. Remember, then, Dr. Selye's advice: "Nature likes variety."

CHAPTER SIX

EAT RIGHT TO SLEEP TIGHT

Your foods shall be your remedies,
and your remedies shall be your foods.
—Hippocrates

The Hippocratic Oath, which dates back to Ancient Greece and the father of medicine, is still recited by new physicians upon completion of their training. Ironically, and perhaps tragically, Hippocrates' injunction regarding food, quoted above, has largely been ignored. Nutrition is rarely a required subject for study in medical school.

"The graduates of today's medical schools know more about heart transplants than they do about basic nutrition," says Dr. Philip R. Lee, director of the Health Policy Program at the University of California Medical School. "I would guess 90 percent of them couldn't describe an adequate, nutritious diet that was appropriate for people at various stages of life."

It may be stretching the point somewhat to say "you are what you eat," but it is undeniably true that diet and nutrition are dangerously neglected in the diagnosis and treatment of disease. That this should be true is ludicrous when we consider the obvious fact that food is, next to air perhaps, our most important source of nourishment and sustenance.

Concern about the inadequacy of the average American diet has grown to the point where Congress is investigating the matter. The U.S. Department of Agriculture has found that most of us consume an alarming amount of useless junk food. In 1970, the average American ate 264 pounds of nutritionless calories—over 50 percent of the total food intake! The number of households with a U.S.D.A.-rated "poor" diet rose from 15 to 20 percent.

Adelle Davis, the late renowned food expert, wrote, "Everything we eat is tinkered with in one way or another. With every tinkering comes losses, some small and unavoidable, some large and avoidable; the cumulative amount of these losses is staggering and crippling."

Since sleep is such a fundamental biochemical phenomenon, it is obviously affected by what we eat. Anyone who has ever tossed and turned to the rumbling of too much pizza and ice cream can testify to that. If what the experts have said about the inadequacies of our diets is true, then many sleep problems might be primarily, if not exclusively, caused by metabolic imbalances resulting from wrong eating habits. Even if diet is not the main cause, it is certainly an important factor, and should be a vital component of any treatment regimen, regardless of diagnosis of the cause.

In our search for nutritional approaches to sleep problems, we had to investigate sources outside the realm of orthodox medicine. We found that expertise is plentiful, although you have to dig some to find it. There is, for example, an entire school of psychiatrists who use megavitamins and nutrition to the virtual exclusion of pharmaceuticals and standard psychoanalytic procedures.

Called "orthomolecular psychiatry," this school of thought has met with a great deal of resistance but is finally coming into its own. One of the founders of orthomolecular psychiatry, and one of its most vocal proponents is Dr. Allan Cott who has been a practicing M.D. since 1936. Dr. Cott trained with the famous Dr. Wilhelm Reich. His distinguished career is marked by his research on the effects of megavitamins on mental illness. He is a Life Fellow of the American Psychiatric Association; a member of the Board of Trustees of the Huxley Institute for Biosocial Research; and President and Founding Fellow of the Academy of Orthomolecular Psychiatry. The following interview was conducted in Dr. Cott's New York City office:

Interview with Allan Cott, M.D.

Question: Dr. Cott, what is orthomolecular psychiatry?

Dr. Cott: Orthomolecular treatment is essentially treatment of illness, or some condition like insomnia, by raising to proper levels of concentration, those substances that are normally present in the body. In this way we hope to provide the optimum molecular environment for the brain.

Question: How did this concept begin? Is it a new specialty?

Dr. Cott: Yes, it's a new direction in medicine, and actually, I think, the most exciting thing that's happened in medicine, certainly in my lifetime, but I think in the history of medicine. It has already come to occupy a unique position. Orthomolecular treatment gives the average person a reasonable alternative to the kind of treatment to which he or she has been exposed.

Question: Has there been much research to support the work of orthomolecular psychiatry?

Dr. Cott: There hasn't been much research to support the exact work we are doing; the application of these nutrients. There's been a very good study reported from the Netherlands by a Dr. Bouzier, in which he reported a positive result in a double blind study indicating that the use of megavitamins in the treatment of schizophrenia is valuable. He produced statistically significant results. There's been some research at the University of Alabama's Department of Neurosciences, which indicates that vitamin B_3—niacinamide—prolongs the stage of Rapid Eye Movement (REM) sleep. In the original experiment, which was done with mice, researchers reported that there was an increase of 17 percent in REM sleep. This in itself was remarkable enough because there are no drugs that can produce that much increase.

Question: Don't drugs decrease REM sleep?

Dr. Cott: Usually. Then they extended the experiment to include human volunteers. They were astonished to find that with one gram of niacinamide taken three times daily for a total of 3,000 milligrams, they recorded an increase of REM sleep by 40 percent.

Question: Were these volunteers people with sleep difficulties?

Dr. Cott: They were college students. But the amazing thing was that they found when they were taking the niacinamide that they were sleeping more soundly, slept less, and felt more refreshed. The electroencephalograph tracing and other things corroborated the fact that they did indeed react as they had expressed. I was delighted that they had documented this in a scientific way. I was not surprised with the results.

Over the years I had been treating hyperactive, learning disabled children who are bright, but can't learn because their brains are racing. One of the things that almost all the parents reported to me was the child was sleeping better. Nighttime would be a nightmare for the family of such a child because he'd be up and down keeping everybody awake and sometimes not going to sleep until he fell on the floor exhausted. These kids began to sleep better with good doses of niacinamide.

Question: Do you get many patients with sleep problems?

Dr. Cott: People who come with sleep problems more often will come with a problem that bothers them even more. Depression. Depression always interrupts or interferes with the sleep pattern. Now and then we have a person only complaining about a sleep problem. When we examine, we do find depression, among other things. We've had good success with the treatment of insomnia. There are many biochemical facets to it. For example, during depression, serotonin level is low. Niacinamide is found in research to enter the biochemical pathway that ends up raising serotonin level. This may be part of the answer to why it helps sleep.

Diet is a very important factor. Poor diet can be involved in depression. People who suffer from hypoglycemia are depressed and fatigued yet they do not get refreshing sleep. They wake up feeling just as exhausted as they felt when they went to bed. When we change their diets, eliminating those substances that over-stimulate the pancreas, like sugar and caffeine and car-bohydrates, which are quickly converted to glucose, they have a more level balance in the blood sugar, and they begin to feel less depressed, and then they start sleeping better. Another thing we find in depression is a high level of histamine. I found that those patients who were having trouble with sleep and who had high histamine levels slept better when I lowered the histamine levels.

Question: These were people who were not necessarily complaining of depression, but were complaining of sleep difficulties?

Dr. Cott: Yes. Or headache. The high histamine level is commonly associated with headache. I've seen many patients who have been to the most prestigious headache clinics who did not get relief until we lowered their histamine level.

Question: How do you diagnose the level of histamine?

Dr. Cott: One, the histamine can be examined in the blood. That is a very expensive test, and the average lab doesn't do it properly. Now we order a lab test called an absolute basophil count. If we find a high level of basophils we can then deduce that the person has more than his or her share of histamine.

Question: How do you treat excessive histamine?

Dr. Cott: Dr. Pfeiffer has reported that methionine, which is an amino acid, and calcium gluconate, which is a min-eral, together lower histamine. It works very nicely without the side effects of antihistamines.

Question: If somebody suspected that he had a histamine problem, could he purchase those items in a health food store or a pharmacy?

Dr. Cott: Any kind of self-treatment for a condition or an illness is not good. People who want to take vitamin and mineral supplements should take them in a balanced form rather than to try treating themselves. For reducing histamine, or helping insomnia, they really ought to consult with somebody who can help them.

Question: If somebody came to you with an insomnia complaint, would it matter to you what the cause was? In other words, somebody might argue that depression causes a physiological imbalance, while another might argue that the physical problem, hypoglycemia or whatever, causes the depression.

Dr. Cott: I don't think it really matters. One should just attack the problem. We find so many of the conditions interrelating. They kind of overlap.

Question: You feel a biochemical approach without paying attention to why, say, a person is depressed, is sufficient?

Dr. Cott: Yes. If a person has a reactive depression to some real event, such as the death of a loved one, there isn't much one can do about that. If a person is suffering from broken sleep during that period then, of course, one would give him some treatment. That type of thing really passes over. But, people come here saying that they just can't go on another day because they've been depressed and have had interrupted sleep for 20 years. We see many like that. We have seen several patients who have actually said they have been depressed for 30 years, and they could document it. Almost half their lifetimes they were in the kind of depression that never lifted fully. They only fluctuated within the depth of their depression, and never completely came out.

Question: And you would ascribe a biochemical basis for this?

Dr. Cott: We certainly look for it. But in many cases even if we did the routine blood test it would not come out much different from a person who is normal. We can't examine for brain serotonin, for example. The closest we could come would be to examine the spinal fluid. We can get some idea, we think, by examining the urine for one of the major metabolites of serotonin. So if a person has low serotonin they tend to be excreting less of the metabolite. But that doesn't always correlate. We just treat the person empirically. Here is a person who has a certain syndrome, which a given number of other patients have responded to with such and such a kind of treatment. We just go ahead and do it.

Question: How would you treat someone if he came to you with some form of insomnia, either failing to fall asleep or premature waking?

Dr. Cott: When they make their appointment they would be given a list of tests that they have to do: an absolute basophil count; a complete blood count; and a biochemical screen on the blood. This gives a base from which to monitor the blood as the treatment goes along. Sometimes we ask for a zinc and copper exam on the blood serum but we get that also from the hair test. We get tissue levels of minerals, and on that we prescribe certain minerals that will help balance things off.

It is interesting how it correlates with a person who has hypoglycemia and who is depressed, irritable and anxious, and has all the other symptoms that go along with the disturbance in glucose metabolism ... they don't sleep well and so on. They will have low levels of calcium generally, and low levels of magnesium as determined in the hair analysis.

Question: Both are associated with sleep difficulties?

Dr. Cott: Yes. There is the schizophrenic patient in whom a disruption of sleep is a diagnostic sign that this patient is relapsing into the illness. The person who suffers from schizophrenia suffers from an overarousal of the brain. His brain is racing, and when he is treated successfully, this racing subsides, stops. I always tell my patients when we get the schizophrenia under control, that the one thing I want them to remember would be to call me the moment they find they are not sleeping well. If we get it early, very quickly, we might, by increasing some of the medication, prevent a relapse. This is another cause of insomnia, and I guess it can almost be thought of as the kind of thing that happens to a person in a tense, anxious situation—they go to bed and they just can't turn off their brain. They're mulling over everything that happened in the day, and they're searching in every direction and interrelating things.

Question: After you do your mineral analysis—the blood test and the hair test—is that sufficient for diagnosis?

Dr. Cott: Sometimes there will be other specific tests we might do, like the five-hour glucose tolerance test. We might also want to see what's happening in the blood serum. And sometimes there are some special urine tests to see if a person is losing excessive amounts of zinc and vitamin B_6. Then we take a detailed history of the symptoms and a detailed account of the dietary habits, and we investigate allergies, because there may be something the person eats that interferes with sleep.

Question: What substances specifically?

Dr. Cott: It can be almost anything—anything might be an allergen for that person's brain.

Question: So, you have ways of testing particular foods. Do you prescribe a specific diet after you've gathered all this information?

Dr. Cott: Yes, we will give the person a very specific diet.

Question: How quickly do you see results?

Dr. Cott: That varies. There are so many variables, one of which is the ability of the body to absorb nutrients. Some people will come and then find it almost impossible to eliminate those foods that we tell them must be eliminated from their diet. They will not understand the importance of that, no matter how much you try to impress it on them. They stumble along and ultimately most of them realize that if they are going to get the maximum help they have to make the maximum effort.

Question: Do many people expect overnight miracles?

Dr. Cott: Some. We tell people that in most instances it is a fairly long treatment. We have some people who finish all the vitamins in the bottle and call up and say, "Well, I've finished all the medicine and I'm not better yet."

Question: It can be very expensive to continue the supplements.

Dr. Cott: Yes, it is unfortunate. The cost of vitamins has gone up tremendously. When we started, a person could buy a thousand of the 100-milligram tablets of pyridoxine for $12. Now a bottle must cost about $40.

Question: Do you monitor the patients so that they can start cutting back on supplements?

Dr. Cott: Yes, we tell the patients that the ultimate goal of the treatment would be to maintain on the minimal amount, and make do with the diet. If they're very ill, we have them check back in a week. We let them know that they can call if they have an emergency. A patient needs a lot of support like that—to be cut off for a couple of months could be devastating.

Question: You mentioned calcium, magnesium and histamine. Are those the factors you generally find deficient?

Dr. Cott: We also find the need for manganese and zinc and vitamin B_{12}. There are very good supplements for these. B_{12} is very commonly deficient. B_3 and B_6 are given, not necessarily because we think the insomniac is deficient, but because these vitamins have an antistress factor. Both have been found to prevent the production of stress-induced ulcers in laboratory rats. Rats are a perfect model for studying the effects of stress.

Question: How about tryptophan?

Dr. Cott: Yes, tryptophan is excellent for sleep. I began doing research with it a number of years ago. We thought at first that this would be a great thing for depression, but it does not work out as well for depression as it does for sleep. I have people take two grams before bedtime.

Question: Right before bed? Does it metabolize that quickly?

Dr. Cott: Yes.

Question: And you've found good results from two grams?

Dr. Cott: Oh, excellent results.

Question: Do you find that you can ultimately cut down from two grams?

Dr. Cott: Yes, but not immediately.

Question: If you had something to say to the people who are reading this book, and who could not consult an orthomolecular psychiatrist or a nutritionist for one reason or another, what advice would you give them?

Dr. Cott: Do not accept Valium as a sleep medication, or use any other type of sleep medication. Try tryptophan; we know it has not produced any side effects.

Question: If a person went to a doctor who prescribed drugs, what would you suggest he or she do?

Dr. Cott: If they've gotten to the point where they are desperate enough to take anything, then accept the sleep medication, but do not use it over the long term. Valium, Librium, or anything that reduces depression or anxiety, will quickly bring about habituation. The wheel gets rolling and the person finds himself taking Valium for three or four years and then he or she can't get off of it.

Question: If somebody wanted to find professional help through nutritional or orthomolecular approach, how would he or she proceed?

Dr. Cott: They could either contact the Huxley Institute for Biosocial Research, 1114 First Ave., New York City, or, the Academy for Orthomolercular Psychiatry at the North Nassau Mental Health Center, 1691 Northern Blvd., Manhasset, N.Y. 11030.

A Visit to a Nutritionist

We wanted to submit ourselves to a nutritional regime under the supervision of an expert to see how it affected our sleep.

By chance social encounter, we met Samuel Bursuk, a consulting health educator and nutritionist for the North Nassau Mental Health Center. Short and husky, well-tanned, with dark, curly hair and an engaging smile, Mr. Bursuk looked like he might be more at home in southern California or Florida than the New York City suburb where he works.

Several years ago, Sy, as he likes to be called, was a "reasonably happy, moderately successful, accomplished, and healthy individual." An engineer and family man, he was, at age 48, suddenly attacked by a set of severely stressful circumstances. Before long he lost his zest; he was depressed, apathetic, and gloomy. He contemplated suicide. And he could not sleep.

He described his insomnia: "As a youngster and throughout most of my adult life, I slept well and was in need of eight hours a night. I enjoyed sleeping. With the onset of my metabolic disturbance, the first thing that happened was a faulty sleep mechanism. I was restless; I awakened unrefreshed. At the height of my illness, sleep was completely broken. Rarely did I get more than two hours of real sleep a night. I would lie in bed for as long as 16 hours a day with my eyes closed, but not sleeping. This lasted nine months or a year."

During that period Sy visited two psychiatrists, an internist, an endocrinologist, and a psychotherapist. Heavily drugged by those experts with phenothiazine and other antipsychotic drugs, including some for sleep, he was eventually hospitalized by what he now calls an overdose. He had involuntary movements of the tongue, arms, and legs. He developed "drug-created malnutrition," and his mental state deteriorated further.

Desperate, despondent, and hopeless, Mr. Bursuk visited—on the advice of a friend—a doctor with an orientation toward nutrition. The physician took a comprehensive medical history, a battery of biochemical blood tests, and a six-hour glucose tolerance test. On the basis of his findings, he prescribed a diet, adding foods to Sy's current intake, and removing some, and he put him on a program of supplemental vitamins and minerals.

"Within seven days, with proper nutrition and megavitamin therapy," says the grateful Mr. Bursuk, "the feeling of depression lifted. Within six weeks I was clear-minded again, motivated, full of zest and energy. And, with the return of well-being, I enjoyed my family relationships and had positive projections of the future."

The last problem to clear up was his sleep. Even when he began feeling better he still did not sleep properly. But when his sleep finally returned to normal, he noticed an interesting change. "I was sleeping less, and sleeping better. I would wake up and bounce out of bed."

He attributes the change in his sleep to a rebalancing of his body chemistry, achieved through primarily nutritional means.

During his illness, Sy was even unable to concentrate on reading a newspaper. After three months of his nutritional therapy, he claims, he was able to read, study, and absorb material. He decided to apply his renewed ability to the study of nutrition. Now, as a nutritional consultant to doctors and dentists, he brings to his work the sort of compassion that only a former sufferer can. He even visits his clients in their homes to get a feeling for their cooking and eating patterns.

To his observations, he adds the responses to a questionnaire and interview, plus optional laboratory tests, some of which the client can administer on his own. Then he recommends a nutritional program.

The first thing Mr. Bursuk does is to steer his clients away from thinking of their insomnia as a disease. He encourages a holistic attitude. "Don't isolate the sleep mechanism," he warns. "Insomnia is a sign, not a disease."

He has worked with about 30 to 40 insomniacs, he said—that is, people whose initial complaint was a chronic sleep problem. But in each case he discovered other, more serious problems that joined with the insomnia to compose a picture of general physiological imbalance. In fact, most of his clients—whatever their primary complaint—had what he called a "disturbed sleep-wake cycle." He claims to have had great success with sleep problems.

While Sy recognizes that psychological and behavioral factors as well as serious organic defects can be involved in sleep difficulties, he feels that the problem can be attacked more or less exclusively through tending to what we put in our mouths.

"The primary cause of insomnia," he says, "is faulty digestion. That leads to deficiencies of vitamins, minerals, and enzymes."

Indeed, that is his feeling about illness in general. "The normal state of human existence is good, vibrant health," he maintains. "Illness and disease are the abnormal conditions."

He goes on to explain that the human organism is a biochemical machine, run by metabolism. If you put junk into it, you will get faulty performance, just as you would if you put kerosene into your car instead of gas.

"If you put in what nature intended," he says, "the body is self-balancing, self-cleansing, and self-healing. When the body is in balance, or homeostasis, it becomes disease-resistant."

With insomniacs, as with most of his clients, he attempts to bring the body back into balance by overcoming deficiencies and stabilizing the metabolism, which he calls the motor of the body. The process that converts foodstuffs into energy, metabolism involves the complex interaction of the endocrine system and the digestive tract. Through that mechanism, the body ingests, digests, assimilates, and utilizes food.

Dietary Solution Takes Discipline

Overcoming insomnia, although a simple matter from his nutritional point of view, is not an overnight process, he cautions. He recalls that, in his own case, the sleep mechanism was the last thing to normalize.

And, he warns, treating physical problems through nutrition differs from the kind of treatment we are used to—it can't be done for you or to you, like injections or medicines. It requires discipline. Without that, the person is not likely to go through the trouble to follow the program as prescribed, and will fall back into old, careless eating habits before the body has a chance to restore its equilibrium. That is a point well worth remembering if you choose to change your diet hoping to improve your sleep. You must be prepared to give it time, and you must stick to it. Don't give up on it, and be strong enough to say "no" when your friends tempt you with forbidden food and tease you about your "fanaticism."

Because we were charmed by anyone who, in this day and age, would make house calls, and because we thought that his status as a formerly severe insomniac would give him a level of insight that another nutritionist might lack, we decided that one of us should become a client of his. Here is the report:

After discussing health in general, and insomnia in particular, with Mr. Bursuk, I filled out a lengthy questionnaire—a "health appraisal indicator"—divided into seven sections: gastrointestinal indications, functional nervous indications, metabolic rate indications, hormone and enzyme indications, fluid balance indications, epithelial indications and carbohydrate indications. Each group was further divided into several sections. In all there were 137 questions, most of which were descriptions of specific symptoms, which I scored "mild," "moderate," or "severe."

In addition, I was to keep a running list of everything I ate for the two weeks prior to our next consultation. I took my pulse rate on arising, before and after meals, and before bed. And every morning I tested my urine for a deficiency in hydrochloric acid. A hair test, designed to diagnose mineral deficiencies, was done later by a laboratory.

At the time of my next meeting, a week after I had given him my completed forms, Sy handed me a large, heavy paper bag. "Here are your supplements," he said. Eleven jars! I was to take them after each meal, in different combinations: 11 in the morning, eight after lunch, and 13 after dinner. The list included: a high potency multivitamin that contained just about everything you can think of; vitamins A, D, C, and E; bone meal, a calcium supplement; pantothenic acid; wheat germ oil and three trophins. It even contained a digestive enzyme because my digestion was determined weak, something I could have predicted, since I was unable to digest protein effectively.

The trophins are enzymes. Certain biochemical disturbances disrupt the manufacture of enzymes that help in digestion, Sy informed me. These trophins are concentrated food substances—raw glandular extracts from animal tissue that become activated in the intestinal tract. Since human enzymes are of identical molecular structure, the trophins help correct disturbed enzyme secretion. He had me take enzymes for the liver, pancreas, and adrenal glands.

He felt hypoglycemia was a major factor in my sleep problems. I found that diagnosis easy to accept. I had been diagnosed hypoglycemic two years earlier, had followed the prescribed diet, and felt and slept much better. Recently, I'd gotten careless, started eating sugar again, ignored critical advice, and found my sleep once again disturbed. I guess I did not want to make the connection, although it should have been obvious, because I did not want to give up sweets again.

The "Allowed" and the "Forbidden"

I was given a list of allowed foods and forbidden foods. The former consisted of good, healthy foods, with an emphasis on fresh fruits and vegetables, and protein—nonmeat sources preferred. In the forbidden category were all the items we love to junk on and feel guilty about afterward, plus several others, all of which are listed in our section on hypoglycemia. In fact, the diet was not difficult to adhere to.

The hardest part of Sy's regime was taking the supplements. There are pitfalls to keep in mind if you use them. Remembering to take them is the first problem. Then you have to overcome the annoyance of the process itself— opening all those little jars and removing one or two tablets, while simultaneously checking your list to make sure you haven't forgotten one, or taken too many of another, or taken the lunchtime combination instead of the dinner. It seemed incredibly tedious. What actually takes a minute or two seemed like hours.

The simplest solution is to set out the next day's pills the night before, making combination packets of each group (breakfast, lunch and supper). Then just pull out the packet and swallow the appropriate combination at home or away.

Once you solve these practical problems, only one remains, perhaps the most significant one. Money. My load of tablets cost me over $50. Some lasted a month, others two or three. If I continued taking them in that dosage, I might have spent $500 a year on vitamins and minerals. At that rate it is easy to convince yourself that you don't need them.

I questioned Sy on just that point. Nutritionists and health food fans are often so enamored of supplements that it is easy to suspect them of the same sort of overzealousness that afflicts M.D. s when it comes to drugs. Sy contended, and most of his colleagues agree, that supplements would be unnecessary *if* we could eat the way nature intended. But our food comes to us long after it is picked, gathered, or slaughtered. Often it is processed, preserved, packaged, and otherwise tampered with. As a result, even if you eat wisely and avoid junk, you will probably miss out on vital nutrients.

In addition, most of us have damaged our digestive systems through years of bad habits before we get around to correcting those habits. Thus, our systems are unable to make the most of what we give them. "It's not so much what you eat," said Sy, "It's what you assimilate. Most people have what we call 'malabsorption syndrome.' They eat like pigs and they don't get the benefits of the food." It's like putting high-octane gas in a poorly maintained engine.

As a result, some form of supplement is probably called for, even for the healthiest among us. Where there is obvious pathology or serious deficiency, large doses of supplements may be necessary to rebuild and rebalance the system. Such a program should be undertaken only under medical supervision. Eventually, with proper diet you should be able to reduce your intake of supplements gradually.

I followed Sy's program as closely as I could. I noticed some changes quite soon—an increase of physical strength, some extra vitality, perhaps less fatigue during the day.

Not all the changes were pleasant, however. I felt some indigestion immediately after eating and taking the supplements. My sleep did not improve, and on some nights was even worse—I awakened with stomach cramps. Sy was not surprised. He attributed this to what he called "the healing crisis." Because of improper digestion, he explained, toxins had accumulated in the system. The enzymes speed up the eliminative process, and the toxins start to be flushed out through the bloodstream. During the period of adaptation, indigestion, sluggishness, or perhaps moodiness can result temporarily.

He suggested that I discontinue the enzymes for a few days to slow down the eliminative process. I did, the symptoms abated, and I resumed at the original dose. This time there were no side effects, and I continued as prescribed.

After four months of relatively faithful adherence to my diet, I concluded that it was probably—with TM and regular exercise—among the most significant things I had done for my sleep problems. I knew this because I woke up less frequently, and, when I did wake up, I found it easier to fall back to sleep.

I feel confident in attributing this change to my new diet for these reasons: I also felt physically stronger; I had fewer battles with indigestion; I did not feel hungry when I awakened; and I had a much less demanding sweet tooth.

The last point is, I believe, particularly significant. As we shall see momentarily, the syndrome known as hypoglycemia can be a major deterrant to natural sleep. It is often characterized by sugar cravings. The change in diet seemed to arrest my hypoglycemic symptoms and stabilize my blood sugar.

When I cheated on my diet I did not sleep as well. That correlation was as clear as day. If I went on a sugar binge (which I did, alas, every few weeks), or if I neglected to eat enough protein, or if I went too long without eating, I reverted back to my previous difficulties.

Our conclusion from this, and the experiences of others, is that nutrition can be the insomniac's first line of defense.

Ideally, anyone seeking to treat insomnia, or any other complaint, through dietary means, should consult an expert like Dr. Cott or Mr. Bursuk. Individually prescribed regimens are, of course, more precise and more reliable.

But professional help is too costly for some and not within convenient distance for others. Many, therefore, look to books for advice. Nutritionists like Adelle Davis, Gaylord Hauser and others, are now taken seriously by large numbers of people. Their books, once largely confined to health foods stores, are featured in major bookstores and at newstands. We combed those shelves for anything that was relevant to sleep and insomnia.

We relied on the most reputable sources, steering clear of faddists and fanatics, and found certain points reiterated over and over again. Only you can decide which of the recommendations best fits your situation. All the advice contained in this section is sound, and can only help your sleep. But beware of making radical changes too quickly. Give your body time to adjust to new habits.

Extract Your Sweet Tooth

Things sweet to taste prove in digestion sour.
—Shakespeare (*Richard II*)

An insomniac musician who is a close friend of ours used to fall asleep all right, but would wake up five or six hours later feeling like his nervous system was "one big, twanging guitar string." Though he was immobilized, he would feel a buzz of activity within. Thoughts raced through his mind as if he were in the midst of a serious business crisis, only they were all disconnected, unrealistic, and irrelevant. His heart pounded furiously. Yet he felt exhausted, unable to get out of bed. He wanted to sleep more.

Basic Pro-Sleep Eating Plan

–Be moderate. Overeating makes excessive demands on the body. Stop eating when you are comfortably full. Don't wait until you are stuffed. Insomniacs should be especially conservative in the evening, as overeating will obstruct sleep. Your body can't rest if it is working overtime to digest a big load.

–Eat only when you are hungry. Trust your body, not the clock.

–Chew thoroughly and eat slowly. Digestion begins in the mouth. Remember the maxim: "Drink your solids and chew your liquids."

–Try not to eat when you are emotionally upset or overtired.

–Favor fresh foods over packaged or pre-prepared or processed foods. Fresh fruits and vegetables are just as easy to prepare as canned or frozen foods, and are well worth the extra time spent shopping for them. Steam or sauté your vegetables—boiling extracts many nutrients.

–Cut down on fatty food, especially animal fats. It is easier to digest fish and fowl, or lean meats, than fatty meats.

–Avoid chemical preservatives, sprays, and additives as much as possible. Studies with hyperactive children have shown improvement, in most cases, as soon as these were eliminated from their diets.

–Avoid, or cut down on sugar and white flour.

Sometimes he would lie in this netherworld of nonsleep and nonwaking for an hour or more before trudging through his morning routine. During the day, he was alternatively depressed and elated, speedy and lethargic, pleasant and gloomy.

The pattern continued until a doctor asked about his late-night eating habits. Upon hearing that the sufferer was fond of sugary snacks, the doctor suggested a blood test. Sure enough, the diagnosis was *hypoglycemia*, or low blood sugar. A change in diet resulted in dramatic improvement.

Whether your insomnia is like the one described above, or you can't fall asleep at all, your blood sugar may be a factor. If you are an occasional insomniac, chances are the nights that you have difficulty are the very nights that you ate sweets or starches in abundance. Check your charts and see.

We are a nation of sugar junkies. According to Drs. Emanuel Cheraskin and William Ringsdorf, Jr., professors of oral medicine at the University of Alabama, "The American eats more candy than eggs; drinks more soft drinks than milk; and downs as much sugar as the combined intake of eggs, all fruits, potatoes, all other vegetables, and whole grain cereals."

Even the conservative *Journal of the American Medical Association* stated in the August 19, 1974 issue that sugar contributes to heart and gall bladder disease, appendicitis, diverticulosis, varicose veins, hiatal hernia, and cancer of the large intestine, as well as insomnia.

Perhaps the most common sugar syndrome is hypoglycemia. Dr. Carlton Fredericks, President of the International Academy of Preventive Medicine, estimates that there are at least 20 million hypoglycemics in the United States. According to a ten-year-old study by the Department of Health, Education and Welfare, "Out of 134,000 people interviewed, 66,000 cases of hypoglycemia were reported. This represents 49.2 percent of those interviewed." It is a good bet that most of us display the classic symptoms of hypoglycemia from time to time, even if they are not so severe as to be revealed in a laboratory. So the information in this section should be useful to anyone looking for ways to improve his or her sleep.

Low blood sugar from too much sugar? Yes. The sugar you consume, and the starches that are turned very quickly into sugar, stimulate the pancreas to secrete insulin, the hormone that transforms sugar and other foods into useable glucose. Too much sugar causes an over-production of insulin, which in turn burns up not only the sugar you have eaten, but some of your reserves of blood sugar as well. This leaves you with too little glucose in the bloodstream, and glucose is the brain's fuel. When it does not get enough glucose from the blood stream, the brain's functions slow down and the victim becomes extremely tired. Normal sleep patterns can be disturbed because the body will react to the shortage of glucose by going into an emergency state. This speeds up certain of your systems, notably the secretion of emergency hormones in the adrenal and other endocrine glands, and that process interferes with sleep.

The usual pattern of low blood sugar victims is to have a rush of energy immediately after eating sugar or starch (when the insulin is stirred to overaction), only to have that followed by fatigue, irritability, and dizziness when the sugar level drops below normal. In severe cases, the symptoms can include vertigo, headaches, cramps, tremors, blurred vision, and cold sweats.

Typically, hypoglycemics experience radical shifts of energy and mood—even during the night, which is why they will awaken frequently, or awaken, as did our friend whom we described earlier, bug-eyed and wired for action. In the long run, the abused pancreas stops working correctly and the symptoms become chronic.

If any of this sounds familiar, and if you have an active sweet tooth, you should check out whether you have hypoglycemia. Your doctor may scoff at the mention of the word. The symptoms are so commonplace, and nutrition is so widely ignored, that dozens of other explanations also sound plausible. It is not uncommon to run across people who go from doctor to doctor being told that they have some psychological disorder or some undiagnosed defect, or just "nervous tension," only to find out one day that they have low blood sugar.

Find a doctor that is sympathetic to your theory and have him administer the glucose tolerance test. It will either eliminate hypoglycemia as a possibility, or it will give you sound clinical evidence that a change in diet is necessary.

The only way to treat hypoglycemia is through diet, and that, ideally, should be adjusted to your individual circumstances—previous habits, taste, weight, and other factors should be considered. However, low blood sugar diets all have certain features in common. Even if you pass the glucose tolerance test, we recommend that every insomniac follow this diet, just to see if it helps:

- Avoid all sugars and sweets. Yes, that means pies, pastries, cookies, candies, sugared breakfast cereals, or your other favorite junk snacks.
- Eliminate coffee, tea, and alcohol. Needless to say, this is important advice for all insomniacs, low blood sugar or not. We will elaborate on caffeine later on.
- Reduce intake of starches. Avoid rice, spaghetti, corn, and potatoes (one or two baked potatoes a week are usually permitted). Limit your bread intake to no more than one slice of whole grain bread per meal (no white bread), toasted if possible. Limit peas, lima beans, baked beans, and cereals.
- Reduce consumption of dried fruits such as dates and raisins.

In addition to these taboos, the hypoglycemic is advised to eat a lot of protein. It metabolizes slowly and will not induce radical shifts of insulin secretion. In addition to dairy products, nuts (especially almonds), legumes, soybeans and avocados are excellent sources of proteins that you can add to your meats or use as substitute for them.

Keep the size of your meals moderate and snack in between. This is to keep the sugar level evenly regulated throughout the day. Two hours after a main meal, and once an hour thereafter have either a glass of fruit juice, a glass of milk, a few nuts, a slice of cheese, or some yogurt. Brewer's yeast is highly recommended with your juice or milk. It is probably better to favor protein snacks over the fruits, but seek a proportion that is comfortable and satisfying.

Dr. Carey Reams, a well respected biophysicist and naturopathic physician, has his patients eat fruits and starches only before 2:00 in the afternoon. "Your body needs energy earlier in the day, not towards evening and bedtime. If starchy foods and fruits are eaten after 2:00 P.M. the energy that's released is not completely used and the sugar builds up in the bloodstream."

Dr. Reams also insists that hypoglycemics get plenty of fresh air and do deep breathing exercises—the liver needs plenty of oxygen to function properly.

Don't fall into the trap of having sugar or coffee for a "quick pick-me-up." You will be quickly put down. Or, your pick-up will come in the middle of the night, when you'd prefer a put-down. If tired, take a nap, and stick to your diet. There are some excellent snacks in addition to the foods described above.

If you ever awaken in the middle of the night feeling something like the insomniac we described at the beginning of this section, it is quite possible that your blood sugar has gone haywire. Take a slice of cheese or a glass of milk. Half a cup of cottage cheese is good if the milk or hard cheese is difficult for you to digest. The added protein might even out the sugar level and allow you to fall back to sleep more easily.

For some people, the knowledge that sugar is affecting their sleep is enough to get them to give it up. Others do not find it easy to resist the temptation, even if the glucose tolerance test and common sense shout it at them. If you are one of these, try this plan:

Cut back, gradually at first, by avoiding sugary and starchy snacks when possible. Eat fruit instead, or nibble on some of the alternatives we mentioned. Then eliminate sugar from your meals, and be vigilant about the ingredients of foods purchased in stores and restaurants because a great deal of sugar is consumed unknowingly. Soon you will find that you crave sugar less and less, especially if you follow the other basic points of good nutrition. We can't help re-emphasizing the value of this for everyone, hypoglycemic or not.

The following interesting facts should help you lean toward healthy snacks: Eating an ounce of sunflower seeds instead of an ounce of potato chips will, in addition to keeping your sugar level moderate, provide you with four times as much protein, four times as much iron, three times as much calcium, nine times as much thiamine, three times as much riboflavin, 14 times as much vitamin A, and twice as much fiber.

So cut down on sweets and have sweet dreams.

Break the Coffee Break Habit

In most parts of the world, coffee is consumed more frequently than any other beverage. Each day Americans consume 400 million cups of coffee. That coffee—and all caffeine products, like chocolate, cola, and tea—tends to disturb sleep through its stimulating effects has long been clearly observed. People commonly take caffeine to keep themselves awake or to "perk up." And those are the same people who commonly can't get to sleep because they are so perked up. Caffeine stimulates the adrenal glands to produce hormones that tell the liver to rush glucose into the bloodstream.

Dr. Weitzman of Montefiore Hospital's sleep clinic related a story to us that is a variation of a common theme: A patient came in complaining of chronic insomnia. It turned out that she drank over 20 cups of coffee a day and didn't realize it until she was asked to count. Dr. Regestein of Peter Brent Brigham Hospital's sleep unit tells of a policeman who would feel alert until 2:00 or 3:00 in the morning. He arose at 8:30 A.M. and went to work. He felt "pooped" on the beat and drank 20 cups of coffee a day in order to stay awake to guard the public safety. He was put on a regular sleep-wake schedule and was gradually weaned of coffee. Eventually, his sleep problem abated.

The case against caffeine has been studied experimentally, always with reinforcing results. According to Karacan et al at the Baylor University sleep disorders center, the systematic study of the way people feel about the quality and quantity of their sleep supports the notion that coffee disturbs sleep. Other studies have generally confirmed that sleep time decreases and the number of awakenings increases when coffee is consumed near bedtime.

According to Dr. Regestein, "The peak of stimulating action may occur two to four hours after ingestion of caffeine, and the duration of the action lasts from two to seven hours. Coffee drunk hours previously may arouse the patient at bedtime. Insomniac patients frequently resort to [caffeine] to overcome fatigue, and this can result in a vicious cycle of caffeine abuse and sleeplessness."

Karacan and his fellow researchers gave different doses of caffeine to 18 normal young adult men a half-hour before bed in a 13-night sleep-lab study. They found that the equivalent of one cup of regular coffee seemed to have little or no effect on sleep. The two-cup equivalent had its greatest effects early in the night (it took longer to fall asleep, and subjects had less of Stages III and IV). The four-cup equivalent, needless to say, affected all measures of sleep in large magnitude. Decaffeinated coffee had no effect on sleep.

The researchers postulate that "caffeine somehow exerts its effects on sleep through alterations in brain metabolites." They also postulate that middle-aged and elderly persons might be more sensitive to caffeine than the young adults tested.

The best bet, of course, would be to give coffee up entirely. Next best would be to confine your coffee intake to the morning hours. What about decaffeinated coffees? Most commercial coffees now come in decaffeinated varieties. However, many health-conscious people object to the additives used in the decaffeinating process, which are suspected of having deleterious effects.

The safest bet, though it may take some getting used to if you are a coffee buff, is to substitute one of the natural grain beverages, such as Postum, Pero, Bam-Bu, or Cafix. They are available at health food stores and in some supermarkets. Kaffir is a pleasant-tasting beverage much like regular coffee, only without caffeine. Herbal teas, of course, are the healthiest coffee substitute.

Some Salty Advice

The next time you are about to shower your food with table salt, consider this: In excessive concentrations, salt acts as a stimulant to the nervous system. It raises the blood pressure by increasing the accumulation of fluids, and it interferes with the elimination of certain waste products of metabolism. It can aggravate insomnia.

Dr. Michael M. Miller of St. Elizabeth's Hospital in Washington, D.C., found that insomniacs whose salt intake was reduced were able to fall asleep within 15 minutes after getting to bed. Most slept through the night. Dr. Miller then restored the salt to 13 of the 25 patients' diets *without their knowledge*. Within a few days, he reports, ten of them had relapses and could not sleep.

While the argument against salt is by no means universally accepted, most health experts with a natural foods orientation seem to be opposed to high salt intake.

Even if you do not accept their judgement, cutting down your salt intake or eliminating it entirely, would seem a sensible thing for someone with sleep problems to do. Your body can certainly do without it. Dr. Mary S. Rose, author of *Foundations of Nutrition*, writes: "The amount of sodium chloride taken in the form of common salt is far in excess of human requirements for sodium and chlorine."

Persons who reduce their salt intake commonly report that their food tastes too bland. Robert Rodale, Publisher of *Prevention* magazine, offers this advice: "Go easy on the salt for a week or two, and your desire for that salty taste will decrease. Only for the first ten days or so of the low-salt regimen will you miss that flavor. Then your taste buds will adjust, and you'll enjoy your food just as much even though you're skipping all that sodium, which can raise your blood pressure and do other harmful things."

When cutting down on salt, try to eat foods that are sufficient in natural mineral salts—uncooked fruits and vegetables, nuts and seeds.

A Juicy Tip

Pure vegetable juice can help restore the proper balance of nutrients in your body. According to Dr. N. W. Walker, author of *Raw Vegetable Juices*, a weakened or fatigued body needs enzymes, the complex substances that enable us to digest food and absorb nutrients. Raw vegetable juice, he says, is an excellent, and quite delicious way to supply those rejuvenative enzymes.

For those with sleep problems, Dr. Walker recommends two full glasses (about 16 ounces) of combined carrot and celery juice at least once a day. The proportion should be nine ounces of carrot to seven ounces of celery.

You can purchase canned or bottled vegetable juices at health food stores. However, if you plan to drink juices on a regular basis, we recommend purchasing your own juicer. Although expensive, juicers prove cheaper in the long run.

Allergies

Most people know that food allergies can lead to sneezing, sinus problems, asthma, rashes, hives, and other obvious reactions. But recent experiments have shown that allergies to such things as milk, sugar, flour or tobacco, contribute to a wide variety of problems, including insomnia.

If you suspect that you are supersensitive to certain foods, try eating more fresh, natural foods—food additives have been found to cause allergic reactions in many people. So have white flour and white sugar.

Find a physician who will give you blood tests and allergy tests to determine what, if anything, you are allergic to. Use your diet chart and sleep chart to see if you can spot a connection between sleeplessness and certain foods.

Some of the recommended natural aids for allergy victims are the same as those described elsewhere in this chapter: calcium, pantothenic acid, and others. In addition, one to four grams of vitamin C per day might be included, as well as hydrochloric acid tablets. Deficiency of hydrochloric acid is a common result of improper diet, and leads to an inability to digest proteins and absorb calcium. Dr. John E. Nelson, consultant to the Council on Nutritional Research, recommends taking hydrochloric acid in tablet form with each meal.

Fasting

Nobel Prizewinning novelist, Upton Sinclair, wrote of his frequent abstentions from eating: "I have found a perfect health, a new state of existence, a feeling of purity and happiness, something unknown to humans."

Actually, the benefits of fasting are far from unknown to humans. *Not* eating is probably the oldest method in the world for restoring health and vitality.

Writes Dr. Allan Cott in his best-selling, *Fasting: The Ultimate Diet*, "No one would dispute the wisdom of getting plenty of rest or taking an occasional vacation. Shouldn't we treat our digestive system to a rest now and then, too? Digesting food is the toughest job our body has to contend with. When we stop eating for a time, we give the system a chance to renew itself."

The body tends to get "clogged up" with waste matter that it hasn't time or energy to eliminate, since we keep adding large quantities of food for it to digest. Like a businessman who closes shop to take inventory and discard superfluous merchandise, the body welcomes an occasional respite from eating to let its eliminative functions get their work done.

Dr. Cott and others have reported excellent results in treating insomnia and related symptoms, such as depression and anxiety, with fasting. In an article on fasting in *Family Circle* magazine, author Jane Howard reported: "Before the fast I used to take meprobamates almost every night, either to fall asleep or to get back to sleep if I woke in the very early morning, as often happened. Now I don't even know where those pills are—it doesn't matter, because I have no more insomnia."

Like Ms. Howard and Mr. Sinclair, fasting enthusiasts tend to wax euphoric on the subject. You usually experience periods of unprecedented energy, alertness, clarity, and well-being during a fast. But, just as likely, there will be periods of discomfort, even pain, as the toxins pass through the bloodstream on their way out. So, approach your fasting with caution and care. Weakness, dizziness, clumsiness, moodiness, irritability; all are possible when you are fasting, and the changes—often from one extreme to the other—occur rapidly at times.

Begin by tapering off. Eat a little less than usual for a few days, replacing heavy foods like meat and starches with fruits and vegetables. Then skip a meal, drinking fruit juice instead. Do this a few times, perhaps three or four days apart.

If you are comfortable with skipping a few meals, you might want to take a longer fast. Approach it systematically and carefully. The books recommended in the reading list are good sources of information. Consult them before, during, and after your fast, and heed their advice. Most of them will cover every contingency, and while they may disagree on finer points, the basics are well understood.

Your first fast should probably be no longer than a day—two days if you are comfortable. Take exercise during the fast—brisk walks are excellent. And drink lots of water to help your body flush out the accumulated toxins that it has been unable to get rid of.

Many experts recommend juice fasts for beginners. At your normal meal times, drink generous amounts of fruit or vegetable juice. This will supply your body with some nutrition, and will make the psychological adjustment to not eating easier to handle.

Many people regularly fast one day a week, either all day or until dinner, with excellent results in both sleep and waking. Some prefer an occasional two- or three-day fast, perhaps once a month. There are many ways to utilize the basic principles of fasting. Do nothing in extreme. If you are hypoglycemic take special care.

Calcium

"Calcium," writes food expert, Adelle Davis, "can be as soothing as a mother, as relaxing as a sedative, and as life-saving as an oxygen tent."

According to Dr. H. C. Sherman of Columbia University, 50 percent of the American people are starving for calcium. Even if exaggerated, that fact could go a long way in explaining mass insomnia in the United States. Calcium has a calming effect on the nervous system. When deficient in this natural sedative, a person is likely to be tense, grouchy, hyperactive, and overly fatigued. Calcium is also important for the proper functioning of the sleep center in the brain.

"A calcium deficiency often shows itself by insomnia," writes Ms. Davis, "The harm done by sleeping pills, to say nothing of the thousands of dollars spent annually on them, could largely be avoided if the calcium intake were adequate. Since milk is our richest source of calcium, warm milk drinks taken before retiring have been advertised for relief from insomnia. . . . For the person whose tissues are starved for calcium, however, the amount in a milk drink is a mere drop in the bucket. I usually tell persons whose insomnia is severe to take temporarily two or three calcium tablets with a milk drink before retiring, and to keep both milk and the tablets on a bedside table and take more every hour if wakefulness persists."

How can we be low on calcium when we ingest so much milk, eggs, and other calcium rich foods? The answer has to do with stress—the same stress that, in other ways, contributes to insomnia. Tension and pressure produce high concentrations of lactic acid in the blood. This acid tends to "bind" the calcium, making it difficult to assimilate.

A quart of milk fortified with a half cup of powdered milk will give you two grams of calcium—the minimal daily amount that Adelle Davis recommends for insomniacs. Cultured buttermilk made from skim milk is said to be an excellent source of calcium, since the acid it contains helps predigest the calcium for easy absorption into the bloodstream. For the sleepless, Davis suggests four glasses of buttermilk daily, along with generous servings of yogurt. (Caution: eating yogurt together with milk can cause stomach upset.)

Other foods to keep around the house: cheese and other dairy products, eggs, figs, oranges, almonds, and calcium-rich vegetables such as cauliflower and broccoli; soybeans, turnip greens, and blackstrap molasses.

Eskimos, who reportedly sleep like babes despite their unfavorable weather conditions, obtain calcium by consuming large amounts of powdered animal bone. You can purchase bone meal in tablet or powder form at a health food store.

According to food experts, our average daily intake of magnesium is about half the adult requirement. If you consume lots of white flour, sugar, or regularly imbibe alcohol—even in small amounts—you are likely to be deficient in magnesium. Magnesium is important for calcium absorption.

Food containing high amounts of magnesium are sea salt, kelp, seeds of all kinds, nuts, beets, spinach, dates, and prunes. You might wish to add magnesium supplements to your diet. According to Gaylord Hauser, "Magnesium oxide supplements taken a half-hour before retiring have replaced the sleeping pill for many insomniacs."

The B Vitamins

Vitamin B_6, or pyridoxine, has been associated with a host of maladies, including insomnia. According to Dr. Richard W. Vilter, author of *Modern Nutrition in Health and Disease*, persons suffering pyridoxine deficiencies will tend to lose weight, and to be apathetic, chronically sleepy, and irritable.

B_6 is known to have a sedative effect on the nerves, and has been used successfully to treat St. Vitus's dance, palsy, and epilepsy. It also seems necessary for the normal functioning of the brain, and is essential for maintaining the proper level of magnesium in the blood, which, as we have seen, is important for assuring normal sleep.

Of special relevance to insomniacs is the fact that, when B_6 is deficient the amino acid tryptophan is not used properly by the body. Tryptophan is the focal point of the latest and most promising research on sleep and is discussed later in this chapter.

Many scientists maintain that almost every American is lacking in B_6, although the requirement varies among individuals and families. For example, families in which several members have had diabetes or epilepsy tend to need larger amounts of B_6. Women taking birth control pills are often seriously deficient. And, according to Dr. Ronald Searcy, the amount of B_6 in your system tends to decrease dramatically with age. With these facts in mind, you might have your doctor administer the simple urine test for determining B_6 deficiencies.

Dr. Paul Gyorgy of the University of Pennsylvania suggests B_6 supplements of 25 milligrams daily to prevent insomnia and similar nervous disorders. Others recommend 50 milligrams daily. If you decide to use a supplement, start small and see how it goes.

Another of the B vitamins, pantothenic acid, is necessary for the proper functioning of every cell in the body. Neither sugar nor fat can be converted into energy without it. It is also a key nutrient for the functioning of the adrenal glands, and is correlated with allergies and hypoglycemia. From our previous discussions, therefore, it is easy to see why pantothenic acid would be a key factor in sleep.

Experiments by Dr. E. P. Ralli of New York University College of medicine suggest that pantothenic acid is never toxic, and that it can protect the body from numerous kinds of stress. A daily supplement of 100 milligrams would be a wise addition to an antiinsomnia regime.

Psychiatrists report that vitamin B_{12} treatments have been helpful in treating depression and insomnia. You may comfortably take supplements of 25 milligrams daily. To determine whether you have a serious deficiency of B_{12} ask your physician to give you a "serum B_{12} test." Your doctor, by the way, may be reluctant to administer tests for vitamin deficiencies, since nutritional treatment has not yet taken a firm hold in medical circles. Be persistent if you suspect you have a major deficiency. And don't be reluctant to take supplements on your own, in moderation, and with the guidance of a good health reference. They are not medicines.

Niacinamide (vitamin B_3) has been known to help sleep difficulties, even in severe cases. This was discussed in our interview with Dr. Cott. Fifty milligrams three times daily has been suggested.

The B vitamin inositol has been used by some nutritionists as a natural sleep-aid. It can be purchased in jars of 100 tablets of 650 milligrams each. Try taking two before bed.

Here is a list of foods that are rich in all the B vitamins: liver and other organ meats; whole grains; wheat germ; walnuts; peanuts; bananas; sunflower seeds; blackstrap molasses. The most concentrated source is brewer's yeast, a virtual wonder food that has an excellent effect on sleep. The authors conducted an informal experiment on themselves, taking brewer's yeast between meals and before bed for a week, then skipping it for a week, then taking it again. We could discern a definite beneficial influence from brewer's yeast on the depth and duration of our sleep.

Brewer's yeast may be obtained in tablet form, or as a powder. It tastes awful to most people at first. But you will soon get used to it mixed with fruit juice (tomato is good) or milk, baked in bread, or sprinkled over cereal. You can buy brewer's yeast at any health food store.

A Word on Supplements

We have mentioned several vitamins and minerals that are known to have an effect on sleep. It would be nice if nutritional imbalances could be corrected simply by eating the right foods. Unfortunately, as we discussed earlier, this is hardly possible. "I take vitamin pills," said Adelle Davis, "and I recommend them, but I still disapprove of them. If wholesome foods were available, supplements would rarely be needed." But, she laments, supplements "appear to be necessary."

When your sleep improves, you may want to start gradually cutting back on the supplements you have been taking to help your sleep. Eat right, live right, and you may not need more than a good multivitamin. On the other hand, it might be wise to take no chances, at least with certain key nutrients like calcium and the B vitamins.

Take your supplements after meals, and spread out the dosage evenly throughout the day, to assure proper absorption.

Ideally, you should consult a nutritionist, an orthomolecular psychiatrist, or a nutrition-oriented physician or chiropractor, to have a supplement program tailor-made for your individual needs. We have synthesized the following list from all those recommended for sleep. If you choose from it selectively—or use them all if you wish—and if you follow some of the simple advice in other parts of this book, you should notice improvement within two or three months if not sooner. Some people notice immediate change.

In addition to eliminating sugar and salt, and drinking lots of milk and/or buttermilk, use all or some of the following, according to your needs:

- 1 strong multivitamin every morning.
- 2 tablespoons of blackstrap molasses.
- 2 tablespoons of brewer's yeast twice a day.
- 2 tablets of calcium, preferably bone meal, with each meal. We recommend 500 mg. tablets with vitamin D and phosphorus.
- 2,000 units of vitamin D.
- 50 mgms. of vitamin B_6 (pyridoxine).
- 25 mgms. of vitamin B_{12}.
- 50 mgms. of niacinamide three times a day.
- 50 mgms. of vitamin C.
- 100 mgms. of pantothenic acid.
- 400 International Units of vitamin E.

In addition, you might consider taking hydrochloric acid tablets with each meal to aid digestion. The glandular concentrates (trophins) that we mentioned earlier might also be a wise investment, especially for severe insomniacs. They can't hurt and might strengthen key organs. Organ weakness may be a fundamental reason for your not sleeping properly. The adrenals, liver, and pancreas are the most likely candidates for weakness especially if symptoms of low blood sugar are evident.

This can be an expensive routine. Without the proper diagnoses, you can't be sure exactly which supplements you need. So be experimental, but don't be too tight-fisted. Supplements are certainly cheaper than medicine, and few people think twice about purchasing that, never stopping to consider the price of the wear and tear on their bodies.

One other supplement should round our our discussion. It is, however, such a potentially important discovery in the young history of sleep research, that it deserves a section of its own.

L-Tryptophan

One of the most familiar folk remedies for insomnia is a glass of warm milk before bed. Not very many people take it seriously, but strangely enough the milk does seem to help. Why? Is it soothing to the digestion, as some suggest? Is it the calcium? Or, as the Freudians propose, is it subconsciously reminiscent of mother's milk?

People have long noted another soporific in daily use—a heavy meal. We tend to collapse in drowsiness after a blowout feast. It was thought that this was caused by blood rushing from the head to the belly, an explanation that turns out to be physiologically unsound.

It seems that the answer to both questions—the warm milk and the big meal—may have been discovered. Milk contains a high concentration of a certain essential amino acid. So do meats, fish, poultry, eggs, dairy products, nuts, soybeans, and other high-protein foods, the very things we usually gulp down in large quantities at a feast. The amino acid is called l-tryptophan, and it is the subject of what many think is a great breakthrough in the search for natural, safe methods for inducing sleep. Many feel that tryptophan may be the long sought-after sleeping pill without side effects. The evidence compiled thus far would indicate that.

Dr. Ernest Hartmann of Boston State Hospital, is responsible for most of the research. "In our studies," he reports, "we found that a dose of one gram of tryptophan will cut down the time it takes to fall asleep from 20 to ten minutes. Its great advantage is that not only do you get to sleep sooner, but you do so without the distortions in sleep patterns that are produced by most sleeping pills."

In a series of 11 experiments conducted over the last seven or eight years, Dr. Hartmann has documented the effects of tryptophan on both rat and human subjects. All the human studies were comparisons of tryptophan, at various doses, with a placebo, under double blind conditions where neither the patient nor the technicians and assistants knew the identity of the medication. Tryptophan and the placebo were administered 20 minutes before bedtime, and records were kept of the usual physiological variables studied in the sleep labs. In addition to being measured for EEG and other physiological variables, the subjects all filled out forms evaluating their sleep the morning after. The subjects ranged from normal sleepers to serious insomniacs.

The following table reprinted from the *Waking and Sleeping Journal* (1977) 1:155-161, summarizes the results of those studies:

Study	Type of subjects	Number of subjects (or patients)	Total nights (after adaptation)	Dose of l-tryptophan compared with placebo	Results reaching statistical significance
1	rats	11	62	150–600 mg/kg	SL reduced at 450, 600 mg/kg
2	NS	10	102	5–10 grams	SL reduced 50%, DT increased slightly
3	MI	10	100	1, 2, 3, 4, 5, 10, 15 grams	SL reduced at 1–15 g SWS increased at 10 g DT reduced at 15 g
4	I	24	192[a]	2, 3, 4, 5 grams	SL reduced ST increased (4, 5 g)
5	I–G	20	160[a]	5 grams	No significant effect
6	I	29	126[a]	5 grams	SL reduced ST increased SQS improved
7	MI	24	96	1 gram	SL reduced DL reduced
8	NS	42	42	1, 3 grams	SL reduced, equally by 1 and 3 grams
9	NS	8	128	1, 4 grams	No long-term changes No changes on discontinuation
10	MI	12	96	1, 10 grams	SL, Waking time decreased (10 g dose)
11	NS	13	—	4 grams	"Sleepiness" increased

SL=Sleep Latency; ST=Sleep Time; SWS=Slow-wave Sleep; SQS=Subjective Quality of Sleep; DL=D-Latency; DT=D-time; NS=Normal Human Subjects; MI=Mild Insomniacs (long latency subjects); I=Insomniacs; G=Geriatric Population.

Dr. Hartmann sums up the results of those studies in this way: "I believe these studies demonstrate that l-tryptophan is effective in reducing sleep latency (the amount of time it takes to fall asleep). This is consistent with [the results obtained by other researchers]. . . . We have also shown that l-tryptophan definitely increases subjective 'sleepiness' in normal subjects.

"There is general agreement that tryptophan reduces sleep latency, and usually reduces waking time; at low doses (1-5 grams) it does so without producing distortions of physiological sleep as measured by EEG recordings.

"Certainly, l-tryptophan should be one of the safer drugs available, since one to two grams are ingested daily in the normal diet. However, an amino acid administered in pure form can produce very different effects from the same amount in a mixture of amino acids and other food substances. Investigations of toxicity after short and long term administration of l-tryptophan is obviously indicated.

"Sleep EEG changes were found neither on long-term administration nor during the month after withdrawal, nor were any psychological symptoms reported during these periods by normal subjects in our studies. . . . L-tryptophan is rapidly metabolized and cleared by the body.

"My impressions from these studies and clinical trials is that l-tryptophan can be useful especially in sleep-onset insomnia and early insomnia. The patients described the effects as an increase in normal tiredness—they were seldom 'knocked out.' "

Why does tryptophan work? L-tryptophan is an essential amino acid that takes part in a number of metabolic processes, including the pathways that lead to proteins and polypeptides. It is directly linked to the production of serotonin, the so-called "sleep juice" that is believed to be related to sleep. Explains Dr. Peter Hauri, "The tryptophan goes from the food into the blood and then to the brain, where it's converted into serotonin." Administering tryptophan has been shown to be an effective way to increase serotonin levels.

Whatever the scientific explanations, l-tryptophan seems to work. Importantly, it is *not* a drug that depresses the central nervous system. It simply fills a deficiency in the same way a vitamin or mineral tablet does, and it allows the body to do what it normally does under ideal conditions. So far, no side effects have been found, even under high doses. In Great Britain, where tryptophan has been used in treating depression, "doses of six to nine grams a day have been taken for a period of many months by several thousand patients with reports of very few side effects and no serious ones."

We gave l-tryptophan to a few insomniacs as an informal experiment, and we took it ourselves for several weeks. It seemed to work just as Dr. Hartmann described. Those of us who usually took a long time falling asleep, fell asleep a bit sooner; those of us who usually woke up prematurely, either did not do so, or fell back to sleep more quickly than usual. One person, who customarily awakened unrefreshed at dawn, took a gram of tryptophan at that time and fell back to sleep 15 minutes later. That, he claimed, was unprecedented.

Of course, we can't rule out psychological distortions in our little experiment; we were all excited by what we'd heard about tryptophan, and wanted very much for it to work, since it seemed to fill all the needs for instant results that sleeping pills do, but without their danger. It is not inconceivable that we all had good results simply because we wanted to and believed we would. That notwithstanding, we did sleep better when we took the tryptophan, and the rigorous studies by Dr. Hartmann and others were designed to rule out such psychological variables.

Dr. Hartmann recommends one gram 20 minutes before bed. Tryptophan is available now in well-stocked health food stores and many pharmacies. You can get it in capsule form—500 mgs. per capsule (two equal one gram). You should also eat those foods that are rich in natural l-tryptophan—high protein foods, mentioned earlier.

Despite the fact that tryptophan has no known side effects, doctors are cautious about prescribing it. Perhaps they recall the many times that new compounds thought to have no side effects, turned out to be destructive in the long run. Also, some doctors are concerned that because of its very effectiveness, tryptophan may be used as a crutch by some insomniacs who might ignore the underlying causes of their problems. Judicious use as needed is recommended; daily use is frowned upon. It will be some time before the complete picture of tryptophan is painted by researchers, but it is off to a promising start.

PRO-SLEEP SUPPLEMENT CHART

Supplement	Effect on the Body	Recommended Daily Intake	Food Sources
Calcium	natural sedative important for nervous system	2 grams+	dairy products, bone meal
Magnesium	natural sedative aids in absorption of calcium	280 mgs	nuts, beets dates, prunes
Vitamin D	maintains nerve health, regulates calcium metabolism	2000 IU's	fish oil, eggs, milk, salmon, tuna
Vitamin E	maintains health of circulatory system, antioxident, reduces toxins in blood	400 IU's	green leafy vegetables, whole grains, wheat germ, vegetable oils
Vitamin B_6 (Pyridoxine)	natural sedative, regulates magnesium and tryptophan metabolism and protein metabolism	50 mgs	organ meats, whole grains, wheat germ, walnuts, peanuts, bananas, sunflower seeds, blackstrap molasses
Vitamin B_{12}	essential to health of nervous system, aids in carbohydrate metabolism, anti-stress effects	25 mgs	yeast, wheat germ, liver, milk, eggs and cheese
Niacinamide	maintains health of circulatory system, antistress effects, reduces tension	50 mgs 3× a day	yeast, organ meats, poultry, fish, wheat germ, nuts, soybeans
Inositol	controls cholesterol maintains health of brain tissue	1300 mgs	beef brain, beef heart, wheat germ, brown rice, brewer's yeast, molasses, nuts, citrus fruit

CHAPTER SEVEN

YOUR MIND AND YOUR SLEEP

How to overcome worry and depression

> The greatest mistake in the treatment of diseases is that there are physicians for the body and physicians for the soul, although the two cannot be separated.
>
> —Plato

It has been over 2,000 years since Plato made that sage remark. Yet, we have been acting as though our minds and bodies could somehow be treated independent of one another. As we stated earlier, insomnia has been handled that way over the years—some see it as a problem of the body; others see it as a problem of the soul. In reality, of course, it is a problem of the whole person.

Most experts recognize this now, but when treating insomnia they tend to put their attention on one side or the other. Most specialists have neither the skill nor the time to gain expertise in more than one discipline. In writing about insomnia, the same problem exists. We can only write about one thing at a time. You, however, are in a better position than either the doctor or the writer—you can treat your insomnia on all fronts at the same time. Remember, therefore, as we discuss sleep from the point of view of the mind, that we cannot disregard the physiological considerations we discussed earlier. Here we shall focus on attitudes, moods, values, the ways in which we handle our problems, and the ways in which we perceive our lives and our sleep.

Often, sleeplessness is a sign of severe mental disorder. Both schizophrenics and manic-depressive psychotics tend to manifest sleep difficulties along with the more tragic symptoms of those diseases. There is little a book like this can do for persons so afflicted, except to say that they should get to a professional mental health expert as soon as possible, meanwhile using this book to help their sleep.

For the most part, insomnia is associated with the classic neurotic symptoms with which most of us are familiar. Through tests and interviews, it has been determined that insomniacs are, as a group, prone to psychosomatic illness, anxious, introverted, hypochrondriacal, and subject to adjustment problems. According to Dr. Quentin Regestein, "Many chronic insomniac patients are described as tense, complaining, histrionic individuals, who are oversensitive to minor discomforts and unable to relax easily."

In discussing the causes of insomnia with psychiatrists and psychologists, we found that there is a wide range of theories to account for the problem. They range from the superanalytical—"Some neurotics feel so weak and vulnerable that they are afraid they will die during sleep"—(Maybe Mark Twain wasn't kidding when he advised, "Don't go to bed, because so many people die there.") to the superbehaviorist—"Sleeplessness is a learned, or conditioned, response to a certain set of stimuli." The recommended treatments are equally diverse.

One of our sources was Dr. David S. Viscott, a psychiatrist with a down-to-earth approach, and a way of appealing to common sense. Dr. Viscott has been a Psychiatric Fellow at Boston State Hospital, and Chief Resident at University Hospital Psychiatric Clinic. He has taught on the faculty of the Boston University Medical School, and served as Senior Psychiatrist and consultant for the state of Massachusetts. He has written several books, among them the best-selling *The Making of a Psychiatrist*, and popular self-help books such as *The Language of Feelings, How to Live With Another Person*, and *Risking*. Here is our interview with Dr. Viscott:

Interview with David Viscott, M.D.

Question: Dr. Viscott, what is your first response when a person comes to you and complains of insomnia?

Dr. Viscott: If a patient comes to me and complains that he can't sleep I ask him "Why can't you sleep?" If you don't ask that question the chances are you're not going to get the most obvious clue because everyone has a reason which is apparent to him and which, if asked, more often than not he'll tell you. I ask "Why can't you sleep? What keeps you up? What do you think about when you're awake?"

You can go into a history of why you don't sleep, but I like to go into the dynamics of falling asleep in terms of what it is that keeps the person up. The chances are the person's coming to you because of a sleep problem that has endured for four or five weeks. For one sleepless night no one's going to go running to his doctor, although some people get needlessly afraid if they're up one or two nights. The stage of sleep that is really threatening to most people is the hypnagogic stage, just when you start to lose consciousness, because in that moment you relinquish your defensive hold on the feelings that are being repressed, held away, isolated.

Characteristically, when people lower their defenses at bedtime their problems seem larger than they did during the day and overwhelm them. So they become frightened and reinstate their defenses and as a result can't relinquish their consciousness, or fall asleep.

There are three kinds of defenses—denial, making excuses, and pretending:

Denial is a primitive response and requires no verbal ability. The denier is in effect saying, "No, Go Away" to his problems. The person who makes excuses says, "I didn't make this mess, someone else did." When such a person relinquishes his hold on his defenses in the hypnagogic state he begins to see the other side of the argument he's been avoiding . . . his blame. And so he has to create more excuses to put the problem away. He loses sleep defending. When defenses are lowered, the denier feels "Woe is me. I can't sleep. Everything is awful. I'm in terror." And the excuser's mind races along reasoning "if I did this or that or . . ."

The person who pretends suffers a similar kind of problem. He pretends that things are the way he wishes they were. He's aware of reality but not its full extent. Unlike the denier he lets more of the pain in, but is likely to turn from it. Most adults tend to be more like pretenders than anything else, although everyone makes excuses, especially when his sense of losing control is overwhelming; people need to make sure that they weren't at fault.

The three major character types, the dependent person, the controlling person and the pretending or competitive person, have their own respective problems. So as each of these people lies down in bed and begins to be released from his defenses, he's likely to be overwhelmed by problems he's not been honest in facing when awake.

Question: What are the problems that overwhelm each of these types?

Dr. Viscott: There are specific problems for each character type. The person who mostly uses denial is usually concerned with a loss of love. The person who makes excuses is concerned with a loss of control. The person who uses pretense is concerned with a loss of esteem. The anxiety that causes sleeplessness is often a mixture of all three potential losses. As a person puts his head down on the pillow his potential losses make themselves known to him.

The defenses that are not effective in containing anxiety in the waking state or in the induction period are similarly ineffective in maintaining sleep, containing the highly charged emotions of the dream.

The dream material embodies and expresses the unresolved emotional concerns of the dreamer. Dreaming is part of the continuum of emotional processing. One wonders if the psychotherapeutic effect of drugs is their ability to allow forbidden feelings to appear during sleep instead of during wakefulness. As an example of how this works, depressed people are helped by expressing the anger which feeds their guilt. It's been shown that in depression, the anger expressed in dreams increases after the use of Tofranil, an antidepressant. Thus troublesome feelings are vented in sleep. Such emotion-discharging sleep becomes a therapeutic process in itself.

Another proof of this mechanism of therapeutic sleep is that patients receiving Valium for the management of anxiety similarly report an increase in the anxiety of dreams.

Each character type has specific issues that concern him. The person who uses denial fears being abandoned. The controlling person fears being out of control. The person who pretends fears being embarrassed by having his shortcomings and pretenses exposed. When one has problems that overload these defenses it will be difficult to stay asleep.

The best approach is to question the insomniac to determine what's troubling him. Define his particular loss (love, control, esteem) and his characterological style of dealing with it. Then help him cope with the fear of the loss directly, without defenses, so that there is less need to defend and less fear generated by relinquishing defenses at the time of initiating sleep or maintaining a therapeutic dream.

Our life is centered around pain and how we cope with it. Losses define everything. When the loss is in the future we call it anxiety; when the loss is in the present we call it pain; when the loss is in the past we call it anger. The question of loss in a person's life, how one deals with a loss, whether one is coping or not, is the therapist's rightful concern. The object is to probe the loss and make it understandable. Sounds easy, though it's not when it's your problem. People in pain are either anticipating a loss, suffering a loss, or reacting to a loss. So they're either anxious, hurt or angry. To resolve their hurt they must feel the loss. There's the fear of losing, the pain of losing, the bitterness and the anger of losing; that's the cycle of the whole human experience of feeling. One must live through the fear, pain and bitterness. Meet fear with understanding, soften pain with time, and treat bitterness with love of self. You have to convince yourself that you are not bad for being bitter.

Question: Can you say something about how an individual can cope with a loss on his own?

Dr. Viscott: To solve the problem of sleeplessness you must solve the underlying problem.

Here is a useful way to approach emotional problems. Any loss will be at one of three possible stages:

Stage I If you fear a loss is about to happen you should try to make a plan to deal with it. Figure out what's going to happen, ask what you can do to alter that. Exercise your judgment so you have the best chance of dealing with the loss.

Stage II If you are hurt, you have to cope with the loss by suffering the pain and trying to keep from losing more than necessary.

Stage III If you did get hurt you're going to feel bitter about it. So you must deal with that anger. You're not expected to be perfect; it's OK to be angry. If you permit yourself to feel it, the next thing you know is you're over it. The process of coping is not pleasant. There are no shortcuts. Some drugs may make you feel a little more comfortable, but usually they'll only slow the process and make you less efficient.

Question: Can most people go through this process of getting in touch with their anger or whatever on their own?

Dr. Viscott: Most people do it on their own. The fact is that most therapy takes place outside the doctor's office, not during the session. Everyone has to get better on his own.

Question: To summarize, then, whatever the cause of the person's insomnia, if it's emotional, it can be dealt with basically in the same way.

Dr. Viscott: Yes, by understanding the nature of the loss and coping with it. That can be difficult because defenses create blind spots. Pretending is one such blind spot. People who pretend frequently see life as a competition with others because they don't want to take responsibility. They fear failure through a loss of self-esteem. People who fear losing control blame others for their mistakes. A person who denies tends to be possessive in his interactions with other people. He gets so involved in relationships that he loses his autonomy, but binds the other person to him in a blind illusion of safety.

Question: What are the worst mistakes a person can make in dealing with the feelings that cause insomnia?

Dr. Viscott: *The most damaging thing you can do to yourself is to hold back unpleasant feelings from expression.* When you do that you divide yourself into a part that feels, and a part defended against feeling; a part that's real for you, and a part that's afraid to be real. The open self says "I feel" and the defensive self says "I fear feeling."

The emotional causes of insomnia are rooted in denying feelings.

Question: How should people approach bedtime?

Dr. Viscott: Don't try to solve your problems then. When defenses are overwhelmed, one's ability to weigh the importance of events and feelings in perspective is lost. To acquire the right attitude for dealing with insomnia, you must understand that you *can't cope with all your problems all the time*. At bedtime when perspective is slanted to begin with because defenses are altered, you can't deal with problems positively. So you shouldn't deal with them at all. Therefore, learn to take a deep breath and say, "I'm not going to deal with this now because I really can't solve it. I'm exhausted, I've had a terrible day and it's not going to get any better by staying up. I can't solve anything between now and the morning anyhow, so I might as well get a good night's sleep." You'll do better with a good night's sleep more than anything else. Don't use this avoidance tactic as an excuse for not dealing with feelings in the daytime; or else tomorrow night will be sleepless too.

Remember, you probably already know everything you need to to solve your problem in the morning. There isn't any fact you're going to find that will change your case. The truth will be the same in the morning. You're just afraid of facing it. You need rest, not knowledge. So take a hot bath or shower, have a glass of hot milk, maybe a shot, brush your teeth, watch some Johnny Carson for a few minutes, yawn, and if you're lucky enough to have a mate who is understanding you may even end up having a good sexual experience. That always helps.

Question: What if you can't turn off your problems?

Dr. Viscott: When you feel guilt over being guilty, anger over being angry, fear over being afraid, and depression over being sad, then it's a problem to have a problem. If you owe a hundred thousand dollars chances are you won't get it tomorrow. So why be miserable by compounding your problems? Just do your best. Don't make having a problem a reason to ruin your life. That *will* kill you.

Your attitude is crucial. It may be corny but it determines how you feel; so, enjoy hyacinths in the spring, listen to Mozart, collect shells at a beach, read a book. Go to the Museum of Fine Arts and look at a Monet. Art and nature help you forget the pain of the moment and to realize that you're part of a greater continuum, that man stands for more than the moment, and that you do too. Do what you can to feel good and also to make things go your way. But don't expect to win all the time.

The problem will solve itself if you experience your feelings and don't lose sleep over it.

Depression

Of all emotional problems, depression is the one most commonly associated with insomnia. Sadness seems to knife its way into sleep in an insidious manner. It is, somehow, more acceptable to a person to lose sleep when angry—venting one's rage at the expense of sleep seems justifiable. But depression just keeps yanking at the bedcovers for no apparent reason, and it seems to run in a vicious cycle—depression keeps you awake, the fact that you can't sleep makes you more depressed, and so on.

The sleep clinic at New York's Montefiore Hospital defines depression this way: "An emotional illness characterized by feelings of sadness, hopelessness, worthlessness, and guilt. It may be mild, resulting from neurosis or a crisis in the patient's life. Neurotic depression is believed to be a 'learned' psychopathology caused by longstanding inappropriate mechanisms of integrating experiences into emotional life. Other forms of depression are severe, and are apparently innate, biochemically and/or genetically determined illnesses."

Dr. Viscott explains further that depression is more than just sadness. It is "a sadness which has lost its relationship to the logical progression of events."

Studies indicate that depressed persons have less than the normal amount of Stages III and IV of sleep. They also have shorter sleep times and more frequent awakenings. Early morning awakenings are associated with endogenous depression, a more or less self-inflicted, chronic state of sadness, not precipitated by any particular outside circumstance.

How to deal with depression? Severe and prolonged cases have too often been treated with antidepressant drugs, a form of therapy that is quickly losing favor. Many, like Dr. Cott, treat depression with megavitamins and nutrition, on the grounds that physiological imbalances, such as hypoglycemia, strongly affect one's mental condition. Then there is psychotherapy, in any of its multitude of forms ranging from classical Freudian psychoanalysis to the newer "growth therapies" that have spun off from the human potential research that has been prevalent in the last few years.

Your local college or university's psychology department will be able to refer you to therapists. So will most physicians. And in most large population areas, there are state or local mental health associations. The American Psychiatric Association has state branches that keep a record of qualified therapists. Several reference books are available as well: *The Directory of Approved Counseling Agencies* gives a complete list of accredited places from which you can obtain therapy. The *Complete Guide to Therapy: From Psychoanalysis to Behavior Modification*, a Pantheon book written by Dr. Joel Kovel summarizes the various options available. For "growth centers" and newer forms of group and individual therapies, write the Association for Humanistic Psychology, 325 9th St., San Francisco, CA. 94103.

Everyone has his or her own ways of lifting the clouds of depression that come to all of us at some time or another. A good movie, a concert, a walk in the woods, a visit with cheerful friends or relatives, and countless other experiences that warm the heart, inspire the imagination, or lighten the mind, should all be seized by the depressed insomniac, especially in the evening prior to bedtime. Choose light, uncomplicated entertainment. Remember, nothing is as uplifting as simple beauty. Nature and good art rejuvenate the soul; they remind you of your roots in the fabric of creation. And they remind you that life is more than a series of problems. They point out that love, joy, and happiness are within everyone's grasp.

At night, select humorous fare, rather than ponderous, intense drama that might keep you up thinking. Kings kept jesters at court for just that reason. Norman Cousins, former editor of *Saturday Review*, was once hospitalized for a serious disease, during which he slept horribly. He had a film projector installed in his room and proceeded to watch Marx Brothers' movies and old *Candid Camera* episodes. "The effect was salubrious," reported the *Prevention* magazine writer who told the story. "Ten minutes of genuine belly laughter gave him at least two hours of pain-free sleep." It also had a positive effect on his symptoms, by the way.

Many people, of course, take great solace and inspiration from their religious traditions. A visit to your church or temple, or a talk with your minister, rabbi or priest can renew your faith in both yourself and the universe. Persons who are not religiously inclined often get the same spiritual lift from contemplating the discoveries of science. Standing on a beach at night, looking up at the distant galaxies, and realizing the immensity of the universe and the corresponding smallness of our earth, is often a good way to put the petty cares of the day in their proper perspective. It may also connect you to the cosmos in the same intimate way that a sermon might connect religious persons to their God. Awe, wonder, and reverence are such powerfully positive emotions that they can often overshadow the most stubborn blues.

We mention these time-tested palliatives even though they might seem self-evident, because they are so often overlooked, just when they are needed most. Persons ridden with cares and woes—most of which are terribly exaggerated—sometimes feel that they cannot afford the time or energy to "indulge" in diversions. They feel they need to weigh their problems at all times, and when they are not doing so they feel guilty of "escaping" or "turning away." Indeed, some experts conjecture that insomniacs often evade sleep because of that same sense of guilt—sleep represents turning their backs on problems. Also, they are sometimes afraid that if they stop thinking about their miseries the solution will somehow evade them.

All of this is nonsense. The mind needs recreation so that it can return to the business at hand refreshed. And return it will, if the problems are real (and if they are not, good riddance). Indeed, the solution is likely to come when least expected. Many a great scientific discovery was made when the scientist left his labors for recreation—the subconcious seems to work at synthesizing knowledge when it is disengaged. The DNA molecule is said to have been conceived when its discoverer, worn out from toil and frustration, decided to stay in bed for a few days. When he was idly cutting out paper dolls, the shape of the molecule flashed—it was a double helix, just like the shape of the dolls as they dangled from his hand.

This is not to advocate escapism. We merely mean to remind you that laughter, beauty, devotion, and love are natural cures that should be employed to their fullest. Escape is not the way to overcome depression or anxiety. Indeed, most psychologists agree that understanding your feelings is vital, and confronting your problems—inner and outer—is necessary for any permanent improvement. "Our sleep," wrote the great psychotherapist, Alfred Adler, "can be undisturbed only if we are free from tension and sure of the solution of our problems."

Learning to manage your inner life intelligently, and learning to deal with the inevitable human problems of loss, fear, or guilt, are of tremendous importance in securing sound sleep. Dr. Viscott, like most psychologists, emphasizes the importance of understanding your feelings. "Nothing influences your life so much as the way you feel," he writes. "So whenever possible you should try to identify your moods. . . . Having a particular feeling doesn't mean that you are good or bad—everyone has angry, sad, or jealous feelings now and then. Admitting your feelings to yourself is the first step in discovering where the feelings come from."

Identifying your feelings in this way need not be painful. It can, in fact, be an exhilarating experience to see your emotions and problems in perspective: why are they there? where do they come from? are they reasonable? are they necessary? Ignoring your feelings can, in the long run, be more damaging than honest confrontation. Repressed emotions can eat away at you subconsciously, and they will keep you awake at night. Moreover, they will not go away—they will just find another outlet, usually with terribly inappropriate timing.

When feelings such as anger or hurt arise, psychologists advise dealing with them immediately, If someone makes you angry, tell him so right away. Most people will be apologetic, and in fact might even be grateful for your honesty.

When you are down, your defenses are also likely to be down, and this could foster honest introspection. On the other hand, you can easily fall into a self-deprecating mood at such times in the name of "honesty." When you are depressed, everything seems dismal, even yourself. So be careful of excessive self-criticism—it too will keep you awake. Honesty means seeing your virtues as well as your shortcomings. And remember, it is not an admission of "mental illness" to consult with a professional therapist at such times. Nor should you be embarrassed to seek the comfort and advice of a minister or a good friend—such persons, blessed with compassion and empathy, can help you gain important insight, and give you a gentle nudge into a carefree sleep.

One major cause of depression is loneliness, which Dr. Rollo May called the "chronic psychic disease of modern man." There are many forms of loneliness, of course, some of which can be overcome with the attainment of friendship, marriage, or just plain good company. But, says Dr. Viscott, "The most important loneliness, the one that only you yourself can cure, is the loneliness for a part of yourself that you believe you have lost or never developed. . . . The best cure for this kind of loneliness is to strive to improve yourself and to try to find satisfaction in doing the things that suit you most. This means taking time to discover yourself and building the courage to face whatever reality you uncover."

In other words, take the time to evaluate yourself candidly. Admit your weaknesses and acknowledge your strengths. Then set out to eliminate the former and accentuate the latter. Look forward to where you want yourself to go and what you want yourself to be—don't dwell on past failures. Take responsibility for both your present condition and your future. Remember that your life is yours to make of it what you will. You are not a helpless pawn in the hands of fate. Blaming your troubles on things outside yourself can be more depressing than self-doubt. Taking responsibility for your own fate can be an awesome burden to anyone who has shied away from it. But, once you get used to it and accept it entirely, you will feel liberated. And, chances are, you will sleep better, knowing that you are in your own hands, and that those are pretty goods hands to be in.

Don't Worry

Of all the negative emotions that sabotage sleep, perhaps the most pernicious is worry. Observe the thoughts that pop into your mind as you lie awake. Chances are, most of them are worries, and in all likelihood a good percentage of the things you worry about are relatively trivial. Some of our habitual worrying can be cleared away by right diet, relaxation, TM, or any of a number of treatments we have discussed, for often physiological imbalances, or general tension, can color our moods negatively. They can make us feel negative about anything we perceive. But we should also attack our habit of worrying.

If you are an habitual worrier, as most insomniacs are, it might be wise to cultivate what Bertrand Russell called "the habit of thinking of things at the right time." Avoid idle speculation about the future, and don't let yourself worry uselessly about the inevitable, or about things over which you have no control. To do otherwise is not only a waste of time, but it will gobble up your sanity and your sleep. Keep your thoughts on pleasant or useful matters. Contemplate a problem only when it is relevant, practical, and all the information is at hand. Once you have taken action and the outcome is no longer in your hands, forget about it. Says Russell, "The wise man thinks about his troubles only when there is some purpose in doing so; at other times he thinks about other things, or, if at night, about nothing at all."

Jane Turner, a schoolteacher, claims she solved her

insomnia by learning how to handle her worries. "I got into the habit," she said, "of sitting down and asking myself if the situation really warrants all that much concern. Nine times out of ten, it does not. Often, the whole thing seems truly ridiculous when examined in an objective light."

Mrs. Turner said that sometimes she required a friend's ear to supplement her own. "I would find an intelligent, sincere, and optimistic person—the more cheerful the better. Somehow, articulating my fears and hearing them as if from someone else's point of view, brought out how very ludicrous some of my worries were."

Worries often arise from vague, free-floating anxiety, or from general dissatisfaction, frustration, or fear. But the mind needs something concrete to attach the feelings to. You can't just worry—you have to worry *about* something. So, you connect the emotion to something, or someone, in your life at that time. Usually, it is not worth the time or energy, for the worry has, in reality, no basis in truth.

In *The Conquest of Happiness*, Bertrand Russell advises: "When misfortune threatens, consider seriously and deliberately what is the very worst that could possibly happen. Having looked this possible misfortune in the face, give yourself sound reasons for thinking that after all it would be no such very terrible disaster."

We do not mean to say that you should develop a blasé attitude, or an ostrichlike disregard for your problems. Nor should you exert strenuous effort to push away negative thoughts. It is very important to keep in mind that any such straining will do about as much to promote sound sleep as a cup of black coffee. If something is weighing heavily on your mind, don't ignore it, step back and look at it objectively. This may first require the sort of mental vacation we discussed earlier—a show, a walk, a concert, or whatever. Then look at the positive side as well as the negative. It is always there if you look hard enough and are prepared to lose the strange security that many people seem to find in believing that the cards are stacked against them. Surely, if you believe they are, they will be. The key—and it is a delicate one—is to learn to balance positiveness with realism.

Richard Wynn, a New York city accountant with whom we spoke, claims to have cured his insomnia by discovering the difference between concern and worry. "I never really understood the distinction," he said. "Finally, it occurred to me that worrying never helps you solve a problem. If anything, it gets in the way of intelligent solutions. To worry is to admit defeat before the battle. I learned to be concerned, in a healthy way, about things that were important."

Instead of anticipating disaster, think back to a rough situation that you made it through, and take inspiration from that. You are stronger and more capable in your worrisome moments than you think you are. Don't think of troublesome situations as problems, think of them as challenges, and as opportunities.

Worry is usually an outgrowth of fear, and many of us are chronically, irrationally, afraid. Afraid of what? Loss of love, poverty, death, illness, disapproval. The tragedy is that, with the exception of death, all other fears are in our control. We act as though they are not, but in fact *we* determine our own losses and gains. Being afraid, therefore, is a waste of time.

It is much more useful to devote your energy to running your life in such a way as to avert the dangers before they come. To say you are afraid, is to say you lack confidence in yourself, in which case the only solution is to build yourself into the kind of person you will have confidence in. If you do that, you will not lose sleep worrying. Remember, great individuals, those who assume great responsibilities, often sleep as soundly as babes. No amount of pressure is enough to disturb their sleep. Why? They are not afraid. They are confident that they can handle anything that comes their way. "I would no sooner lose to insomnia," said a football coach who was known to fall asleep on busses and in the locker room, "than I would to a rival football team."

Truly, as Franklin D. Roosevelt said, "we have nothing to fear but fear itself." Our subconscious mind works with what we feed it. In the words of Napoleon Hill, whose best-selling *Think and Grow Rich* has inspired millions of readers, our subconscious "will translate into reality a thought driven by fear just as readily as it will translate into reality a thought driven by courage or faith."

Give your mind more desirable, positive thoughts on which to feed. When you find yourself overwhelmed by fear, jealousy, hatred, greed, or anger, it is your responsibility to yourself to look at the brighter side. Whether we see the bright or the gloomy depends on a lot of things—Our health, our circumstances, our friends, and so on—but it also is a matter of habit. Many of us have caught the spirit of pessimism that has gripped the modern age. We have come to accept disappointment and frustration as inevitable. That is nonsense. Thinking they are inevitable will make it so. But thinking they are unnecessary, and that happiness is your birthright, will make *that* inevitable. Cultivate the habit of thinking positively—replace the negative with faith, love, hope, reverence, and devotion. Once the habit is developed it is as easy as switching channels on a T.V.

You must, of course, not try to drive positive thoughts into your mind forceably. That will only give you a headache, which will probably keep you up nights. Be gentle and patient—old habits are not broken easily. Nor should you fall into the trap of "mood making." Don't go around with a blissful countenance when everything around you is collapsing. Don't pretend that problems don't exist. Just train your mind to see the positive side, and to replace the gloomy with the bright when it is not necessary to be thinking about your problems.

"Kill the habit of worry, in all its forms," advises Mr. Hill, "by reaching a general, blanket decision that nothing which life has to offer is worth the price of worry. With this decision will come poise, peace of mind, and calmness of thought which will bring happiness." And, we must add, sound sleep!

There is one thing that every insomniac worries about more than anything else. It happens to be the one worry that kills more sleep than any other worry. It also happens to be the one worry that least deserves to be a worry. We are referring to the tragic habit of worrying over sleep.

Don't Lose Sleep Over Losing Sleep

Herbert Spencer, the nineteenth century philosopher, once lived in a boarding house, where he would aggravate his fellow tenants with constant complaints about his sleeplessness. He was so obsessed with his problem that he took opium to induce sleep, and used earplugs and other devices. One night he shared a room with a professor friend of his. In the morning, Spencer declared, as usual, that he hadn't slept a wink all night. "Neither did I," replied the professor, "Your snoring kept me awake."

Spencer was not the only one to suffer from what is called *pseudoinsomnia*. Every sleep expert has at least one good story to offer. Says Dr. Richard J. Wyatt of the National Institute of Mental Health, "All physicians are aware of subjective complaints of patients who report that they haven't slept for days or months. When these same patients are hospitalized and are under the scrutiny of a nursing staff checking for sleep throughout the night, it is invariably reported that the patient is in fact sleeping . . . and for long periods."

Dr. William C. Dement, pioneer sleep researcher at Stanford University, says that, "Although *every* insomniac came to our clinic as his 'last hope' in getting some respite from the tortures of sleeplessness, the severity of their complaint had *absolutely no relation* to the amount they slept in the laboratory."

He and his colleagues related this story in the December, 1975 issue of *Psychology Today*:

"A real estate broker, Barry G. . . . . had been forced into early retirement, he told us, by loss of sleep at night and a consequent fatigue during the day. He reported that each evening he lay awake an hour or more, then woke up uneasily several times in the night and could never sleep beyond 5:00 o'clock in the morning. He averaged less than five hours a night, he said, and his wife told us that he was obsessed with the need to get 'his proper sleep.' He got no relief from pills or psychiatry. When we asked him to keep a diary and to record his daytime feeling of sleepiness every 15 minutes, he confirmed his complaints in great detail.

"But when he came to the clinic for two all-night sleep recordings, his body told a very different story. He was a normal sleeper. He actually fell asleep in less than ten minutes and was awake for only 20 minutes all night. He spent seven hours and 13 minutes in normal sleep."

Often, a person who confronts the fact of his pseudoinsomnia by seeing the evidence in the sleep clinic needs nothing more. The patient described above sent the Stanford clinic this letter three months after he was told he slept normally:

". . . Now that I know that I get a normal amount of sleep

I don't fret and worry about sleeping. I seem to awaken less frequently during the night. It is a relief not to use sleeping tablets any more, as they made me dopey and depressed. I find that nowadays I am not particularly depressed."

He discovered what many others have: worrying over sleep loss can be a better means of losing sleep than encouraging the pounding of a pneumatic drill outside your bedroom window. Psychologists have coined a word for it—*agrypniaphobia*, a somewhat pretentious word that means, simply, fear of insomnia.

But why do people think they don't sleep when they actually do? So-called "poor sleepers" have been found, statistically, to underestimate the actual time spent sleeping far more than "good sleepers."

One reason might be a form of hypochondria. Some people have a need to have something wrong with them. Why not invent insomnia?

Gay Gaer Luce, author of *Insomnia*, suggests that "the sleeper remembers only the last stage of sleep, when he is close to awakening. Thus, although the lab monitors that he slept six hours, he thinks he slept only 20 minutes. Or it may be that all of the person's sleeping is spent in a very light stage of sleep."

Some People Dream They Are Awake!

Another theory is that the persons may be sleeping perfectly normally, but *dream* they are awake. Dr. Peter Hauri of Dartmouth tells the story of a student who came to his lab complaining that he could not sleep. In the clinic, it was determined that he slept a full eight hours. Yet, he was exhausted by morning. Analysis revealed that he had been dreaming he was not asleep.

Whatever the reason, you may, in fact, be getting a lot more sleep than you think you are. Persons who toss and turn a great deal are likely to turn minutes into hours in their imaginations. Experts agree that even long periods of night-time wakefulness are punctuated by brief periods of genuine sleep.

Another reasons not to fear insomnia is that you may simply need less sleep than you think you do. We have all grown up under the misconception that everyone should get eight hours of solid sleep a night. Not so. There is no rule as to the proper length of time that any one of us should sleep. According to a 1962 survey, 61 percent sleep the customary eight hours, 23 percent sleep less than eight (with 8 percent sleeping less than five hours) and 15 percent sleep at least nine hours.

Dr. Hauri tells the story of a 70-year-old woman "whose husband sent her to the clinic because he thought she had a sleep disorder: she only slept four hours a night. She told me that she hadn't ever slept much more than four hours a night in her whole life—she thought it was peculiar too.

"Well, we tested her in the laboratory, and there was nothing at all wrong. What she did have was a remarkably efficient sleep. She went very quickly into deep delta slumber, the Stage III and IV phases. And then, after about an hour and a half of that, up she came. She went directly into a little REM dream period. After that, back down she went, came out once more, and then it was all over. And if she didn't have more than a tiny bit of the Stage I or Stage II intermediate stuff, it was because she didn't actually need more than the four hours of sleep. She was as sound as a bell."

How much sleep do you need? Only you know. Some have been known to do with very little, among them Napoleon, Edison, Churchill, Gladstone, and Goethe. The great architect and philosopher, R. Buckminster Fuller slept only four hours a day—in half hour naps every three hours around the clock. He thrived on that schedule until he had to give it up because he was too out of tune with the rest of us.

Than there are the unverified claims of exceptional people, like some of the yogis of India, who, it is said, need barely any sleep at all. The record for verified short sleep belongs to two Australian men, aged 30 and 54, who needed less than three hours a night. The *Guinness Book of World Records* notes the case of Mr. Valentine Medina, a 75-year-old Spaniard who farms by day and patrols his village by night. He claims to have lost all desire to sleep in 1904 and has not slept since. Says Señor Medina, "I've taken sleeping pills until I rattle, but it does no good."

Guinness also records the longest period of voluntary sleep deprivation: 282 hours and 55 minutes (over 11 days), a record held by Mrs. Bertha Van Der Merwe, a South African housewife, aged 52 at the time. An American high school student named Randy Gardner stayed awake, with a little help from his friends, for 264 hours and 12 minutes. Randy had broken the record of Peter Tripp, the New York disc jockey whose 200-hour publicity "wakathon" we mentioned earlier.

On the other side of the coin are long-sleepers, such as comedian-musician Steve Allen. Mr. Allen has managed to write 17 books and 4,000 songs in addition to his television performances. Yet he sleeps 11 hours a night. To make up for lost time he keeps a pencil and pad at his bedside. Reportedly, his biggest hit, *"This Could Be the Start of Something Big,"* came to him in a dream.

There are several lessons in these cases, each of which should help you to cut down on the amount of worrying you do over what you think is insomnia. First, all of the studies on sleep deprivation have shown that people recover astoundingly well, even from severe deprivation. "One thing we have learned," reports British psychologist, R.T. Wilkinson, "is that if people *want* to maintain normal performance, it's surprising how well they can." He was referring to the insomniac's ability to perform as expected following a bout with sleeplessness.

Researchers have found a definite correlation between physical and emotional strength and a person's ability to recover from sleep loss. Highly motivated, confident, healthy people perform better following an interrupted night's sleep than do the chronic complainers, the worriers, and the insecure. Remember then, if you want to function well, you will, despite having lost sleep. Knowing that insomnia need not devastate you should cut down on the anxiety that will, by creating a vicious worry-go-round, keep you awake again the next night.

Another lesson to learn is not to force your sleep pattern into some arbitrarily preconceived notion of how long you should sleep. Determine your own natural sleep requirement and your most efficient pattern, and use that as your yardstick. Your own inner rhythms may be different from the pattern implanted in our minds and on our routines by social customs. We respect individuality enough to accept the fact that some of us eat less, or more, than others, and that we do so at different times. We also have different requirements for exercise, entertainment, money, and everything else. Why not for sleep?

There are many people who think they are insomniacs because they can't get to sleep "on time." Richard Campbell, a 56-year-old lawyer, thought for years that he had insomnia. He would get to bed at 11, and proceed to toss fitfully for two to three hours, feeling wide awake. In the morning, he would struggle out of bed with the alarm reverberating in his cloudy mind, and trudge off to meet a client at 9:00. After some time of this, he took sleeping pills, only to discover the side effects we have discussed. He did not know what to do. Then a passing remark from a friend changed his life: "Why don't you just stay up?"

Mr. Campbell never had heard such a sensible remark. He started to go to sleep when he felt tired, not when the clock read 11:00. He fell asleep within minutes every night. Of course he woke up later as well, something that took some weeks to get accustomed to. Soon, he rearranged his whole schedule, never making appointments before 10:00 unless he absolutely had to. He felt much more productive, used his late hours intelligently, and all in all, made much better use of his 24-hour day.

The reverse is also quite common. Betty Nichols, a schoolteacher from Boston, used to awaken around dawn, never fully refreshed. She would lie in bed until she was forced out by the need to make breakfast for her children, and then proceed exhausted to school. It turned out that at night Mrs. Nichols would stay up at least until Johnny Carson had finished his monologue, and longer if she was attracted by his guest stars. One week Mr. Carson was on vacation and his substitute did not appeal to Mrs. Nichols at all. "I think I'll take the opportunity to get to bed earlier," she thought. It took only three days to get used to it. Then she hit the hay at 9:30, slept soundly, and woke up at dawn as usual. But now she woke up refreshed.

Mrs. Nichols' internal clock was geared to an early-to-bed-and early-to-rise routine. She no longer trudged through the day, and she made excellent use of those fresh, early morning hours when everyone else was asleep. Of course, she missed Johnny Carson, but she soon got over that.

Better to Sleep in Separate Stages

Some of us are better suited to a *polyphasic* pattern of sleep, meaning that we would be better off sleeping in separate stages rather than in one long one. Some people get fed up with their nighttime awakenings, and just get up and do something constructive. They go back to sleep when they feel the need, and usually take a nap or two during the day.

Dr. Roger Williams, professor of biochemistry at the University of Texas, describes something like that in his book *You Are Extraordinary*: "I do not regard my condition as a disease; if it is, it is an attractive one for me. My mind is clearest during this hour or so and I reserve this time to do my best thinking. I go to bed with problems unsolved, but when I get up in the morning after having had this quiet hour in the night, the best solution I can devise inevitably comes to me."

Unfortunately, the requirements of your business, profession, or family life, may not enable you to adopt so individual a pattern. The persons we mentioned were fortunate enough to be able to adjust their sleep to their own needs. Do the best you can. If, for example, you must be at work early in the morning when you are, by nature, a late sleeper and a late riser, you might have a talk with your boss. Explain that you will make up the time in the evening, and that you predict your productivity will skyrocket. Perhaps someday, society will come to appreciate the need for proper sleep, and differences will be accommodated more hospitably.

In determining whether, in fact, your sleep problems are really worthy of concern and not something easily adjusted to with proper understanding or a new schedule, keep in mind that your sleep needs vary with circumstances. For example, we need more sleep during periods of crisis or change, and during emotional or psychological strain. Women may need more sleep during pregnancy, or during their menstrual period. They may, at those times, also experience temporary insomnia. Your sleep problem may only be temporary. During periods of crisis, insomnia is common.

A sudden change in your work schedule, new or irregular shifts, working overtime, or even a sudden round of evening entertainment can cause a temporary problem with sleep. So may a sudden change in diet, especially if the change includes a lot of sugar or stimulants. Of course, the increasing phenomenon of crossing time zones is a common cause of temporary sleep loss.

As You Age You Sleep Less

It is extremely important to understand that your sleep needs tend to diminish with age. If you suddenly find yourself sleeping less, it may not be cause for concern, but the natural effect of aging. "Nothing else changes so measurably between the ages of 20 and 50 as sleep," says Dr. Irwin Feinberg of the Fort Miley Veterans Administration Hospital in San Francisco. "Deep sleep is reduced by 60 percent. The number of arousals in the night doubles. People over 70 spend more time in bed, but less time asleep. Their sleep is constantly fragmented, disturbed by awakenings."

Dr. Feinberg's statement is echoed by every sleep expert. Montefiore Hospital's sleep clinic reports this pattern: "Sleep efficiency decreases after 30 years in men and 50 years in women, then decreases more steeply in both sexes after the mid-50s. The number of awakenings per night increases gradually until 40 years in men and 70 years in women, then increases more steeply after those ages."

Just knowing this, and allowing themselves the well-earned privilege of napping as often as they need, has kept many older persons away from sleeping pills. "People who get older need less sleep," says Dr. Milton Kramer, professor of psychiatry at the University of Cincinnati, "but because they've been raised on the myth of 'a normal eight hours sleep,' they're likely to be the first customers for all those sleeping pills on the market that end up doing more harm than good."

Another thing to be aware of is that waking frequently at night is relatively normal, especially in older people. According to Dr. Hauri, adults generally awaken three to five times during a healthy night's sleep. Most people return to sleep instantly, and do not remember having awakened. It is those who do remember that often get alarmed unnecessarily. If you find yourself aroused at night, the only important questions to ask are: "Does it take excessively long to fall back asleep?" and, "are you tired during the day?"

Just knowing these facts may eliminate many readers from the category of insomniacs. We hope that is true. If you are still doubtful, there are certain key factors that you should consider. Determining whether or not your sleep is problematic requires more than a clock. According to Luce and Segal, authors of *Insomnia*, these are the questions you should ask yourself: how dramatically has your sleep changed? how long have the disturbances lasted? how severe are the attendant signs of emotional instability and loss of efficiency? If the change has been dramatic and persistent; if lethargy, irritability, poor coordination, lapses of attention, and other side effects are excessive, you have good reason to be concerned.

But you still have no reason to be worried.

Even if your insomnia is genuine, it is easily cured. You need nothing more than, well, a good night's sleep. And that is probably easier to get than you think. This book provides you with the complete range of natural ways to induce sleep. If none of them work, the book will explain how to get competent professional help. Your body will simply not tolerate sleeplessness for too long, just as it will not tolerate hunger. Somehow you will find your way back to healthy sleep, if you are determined.

Until we reach that point here's another thought to comfort you and help you not bemoan your sleeplessness too much: it could be worse. When F. Scott Fitzgerald wrote, "The worst thing in the world is to try to sleep and not to," he may have failed to consider the opposite situation: the person who wants to be awake but sleeps instead.

Studies have shown that people with *hypersomnia* suffer the same sorts of difficulties that insomniacs do. But the poor things don't even get to enjoy being awake. At least insomniacs have time to read.

To sum up, it is wise not to worry about losing sleep. We

gave you many reasons why that is so, the most important of which is that the worrying will be self-fulfilling.

If all our reasons fail to stop you from worrying about your sleep, pin up this terse reminder by sleep expert, Dr. Nathaniel Kleitman: "No one ever died of insomnia."

CHAPTER EIGHT

HOW TO COURT SLEEP AT BEDTIME

Sleep is the most moronic fraternity in the
world, with the heaviest dues and the crudest
rituals.

—Vladimir Nabokov

Sleep is the one fraternity to which we would all like a
lifetime membership. So far, most of our discussion has
centered on ways in which to overcome the physical and
psychological reasons why so many of us have been black-
balled from the club. In previous chapters our suggestions
have dealt largely with things to do during the day—ways to
improve your mental and physical health. But now we are
getting on to nightfall, and we must address ourselves to the
best ways to prepare for sleep.

Some of those "rituals" to which Mr. Nabokov referred
can be pretty bizarre. Sleep researcher Gay Gaer Luce
describes a man who paints his face white and goes to sleep
in a coffin. "He has a thing about death," said Ms. Luce, "and
the only way he can resolve it is to actively play dead."

Others are less weird, but still humorously idiosyncratic.
Van Gogh insisted he could only sleep on a pillow made of
hops, a ritual that actually has a long history in folklore. Abe

Lincoln always took a long midnight walk. Catherine the Great would never go to sleep without having her servants brush her hair 100 times.

We all have our own rituals, some elaborate, some so simple as to hardly justify the word ritual. Yet even the simple ones are indispensable—you don't feel quite right about hitting the hay—or hops—without them. If you don't believe you are dependent on pre-bed rituals, try sleeping in a strange place where you can't follow your customary routine. Try going to bed without brushing your teeth, for example, or without watching the late news, or reading, or locking the door, or without pajamas, or a goodnight kiss, or a glass of whatever it is you're accustomed to.

If you do not have identifiable rituals, that may be part of your problem. Maybe you need to find some that work for you and make them a habit. On the other hand, perhaps some of your established rituals are not good ones and are actually interfering with your sleep. There is no universal formula, of course, but there are certain features that good rituals should have. In this chapter, we will discuss the proper way to treat your evening activities and your environment to induce sleep.

Actually, the word "induce" is probably the wrong choice. "The idea of 'inducing sleep' is absurd," wrote Arnold Bennett. "Sleep ought not to have to be enticed like a frightened fawn. It should pounce on you like a tiger."

True enough, but why not do all we can to bait the trap?

Winding Down

You should start preparing for bed long before your actual bedtime. Dr. Dean Foster, consultant to the Sleep Research Foundation, once wrote, "Going to sleep is like stopping a car at an intersection. A driver who sees a traffic light change a block away is better off slowing down gradually and coasting to a stop, rather than coming to a sudden brake-slamming halt. Taper off your day's activities before getting ready for bed."

In our chapter on stress, we reminded you to leave your work at the office. Start winding down when you get home. That is your time to jog, meditate, take a walk with your spouse and children, or read the newspaper; if you have troubled sleep, it is *not* the time to worry about the next day at work or to review all your problems. If your work is so aggravating that you consistently can't get it off your mind, you should seriously consider whether or not it's worth it. Either get a new job, or learn to leave it behind you.

If you must bring paper work home with you, do it early in the evening, or stop at least an hour before bedtime. Your late-night reading should be light, and not call for concentrated thought. Read things that are completely unrelated to your work. Read fiction, but not the sort that is so gripping that you won't be able to put it down, or it will keep you up wondering what is going to happen next. Read to a logical stopping point, leaving no loose ends.

Professor Edward Bauer, a psychoanalyst who used to have trouble falling asleep, claims to have solved his problem by switching reading matter. "I used to read the case histories of my next day's patients before bed," he said. "But it was so stimulating, and it got me so worked up planning how I was going to deal with these troubled people, that I couldn't fall asleep. Finally, I took to reading the histories on the train going home, devoting the rest of the night to recreation. I still have to read before bed, but now I read detective stories. I've been through all of Sherlock Holmes twice, and I sleep like a baby."

Another person whose reading habits changed his sleep was John Wagner, who is in charge of publicity at a major publishing house. "I like to read in bed," said John, "but I used to read the works of the authors that we were working with. It got me thinking too much about publicity campaigns." A religious man, Mr. Wagner switched to his favorite theologian, Thomas Merton. "I fall asleep soothed and inspired by a great man's words," he says.

Religious works are often favored by people who read themselves to sleep. It is more than superstition, and more than the fervor of the Gideon Society that makes the Bible a common fixture on end tables. For spiritual persons nothing is more soothing, or more elevating than inspirational writings.

Your choice of reading matter is, ultimately, a matter of taste. But before sleep, choose those things that are pleasantly interesting, saving the gripping and demanding for other times. Poetry is a safe bet, especially lyrical works. You can't miss with Shakespeare, but stick to the comedies and sonnets; avoid sleep-robbers like *Macbeth* and *Othello*.

The worst thing to read right before bed is anything about insomnia. It is sure to keep you up thinking and worrying about your sleep. And remember, if you do read in bed, keep your lamp at your bedside so you don't have to get up to turn it off.

So much for reading. What about other nighttime entertainment? The same rules apply. If you are a movie fan, or a theater buff, or a TV watcher, try to keep it light as you approach sleep time. Go to early movies if you insist on heavy drama or violence, and take the time to wind down thoroughly afterward. Better still, keep your thought-provoking or titillating fare for weekends when you can make up for being unable to get to sleep on time. During the week, keep it fun and simple. Perhaps you might lean toward music instead of drama.

One of our friends, a businessman named Arthur Kaplan, always had trouble sleeping on Monday nights. For a long time he thought it was because Tuesday was the day of his weekly staff meeting, an event that he had come to dread. When his meetings were switched to Thursdays, he assumed that he would then have trouble sleeping on Wednesday nights. Not so. Monday was still the bad night. Then he discovered the reason: Monday night football. He tossed and turned to the memory of Howard Cosell's commentary, and he replayed all the big plays in his mind's eye. It was not easy to break the habit, but when he decided to limit his football viewing to Sunday afternoons, Mr. Kaplan slept a lot better.

Several sports fans admitted to a similar fate with evening spectatorship. They all noticed the same thing—when their team won, they slept well; when their team lost the game, they lost their sleep.

Even your conversations will affect your sleep. Don't invite guests with whom you are likely to get into a late-night argument. End your social events early, unless you are just plain having fun. Stimulating discussions can keep you thinking after the lights are out. Nighttime arguments are lethal to an insomniac. If you have a bone to pick with your spouse, pick it early. That will give you lots of time to calm down, forgive, forget, and make up, before going to bed.

Regularity

Just about every authority on the subject recommends—indeed, insists on—regular sleeping habits. Find through experiment the most efficient time for you to get to sleep, and stick to it. If further experimentation is necessary, try each alternative bedtime for two weeks, to give it time to establish a rhythm. If you find a set of rituals that seems to create the proper mood and atmosphere for sleep, stick with it every night. The nightly repetition will help you to gain sleep habits that will become involuntary and effortless.

Once you establish a bedtime, be ready for it well in advance. Joan Black, an insomniac college student who was ordered by her doctor to be in bed by 11:00 found after two weeks that it had made no difference. She would wait until the last possible moment before dropping her studies. Then she would dash into the bathroom, brush her teeth, hurry to the bedroom and quickly undress. She practically dove into bed just under the wire every night. Then she wondered why it took an hour to fall asleep.

Better to be early into bed than late. Perform your ablutions and rituals in a leisurely manner. And while you're preparing for bed in that way, turn your thoughts to pleasant memories of the day, or to anything else that makes you feel good. That is *not* the time to plan tomorrow.

What time should you go to bed? Obviously, that is an individual matter. If you seem to have a choice, it's a good idea to opt for the earlier time. The old adage about "early to bed and early to rise," may have more to it than its catchy rhyme. "One hour's sleep before midnight is worth two after," wrote Henry Fielding. It has been echoed many times. There might be something to it.

A study by Johns, Dudley, and Masterson at an Australian university, noted that "better academic performance as a medical student has been shown to be related both to early morning awakening and to better mental health."

For a more scientific method of selecting your best time, try going by your temperature. It has been found that a person's body temperature drops at night, and according to one science writer, that's a signal to the body and mind that it's time to go to sleep. You might take your temperature several times during the evening to pinpoint the time when it drops.

Probably the best way to determine your maximal opportunity for sleep is simply to listen to your body. It knows best. When the yawns come, when the mind starts to wander, when you find yourself reading every paragraph twice, when you can't tell the difference between the program and the commercials, then it's probably time to shut your eyes for the night. Don't make the mistake—a common one that keeps many awake—of fighting it. Forget about the climax of the show—let your spouse fill you in the next day. If you fight to stay awake you are likely to win. And the effects of that little victory will linger—you won't be able to sleep half an hour later either. Your body will have mobilized its energies to meet your demands, and will not be able to retreat so easily.

Snacks and Nightcaps

The great actress Marlene Dietrich says that the only thing that helps her sleep is a sardine-and-onion sandwich on rye. Teddy Roosevelt was lulled to sleep by a shot of cognac in a glass of milk.

We can't say whether or not sardines or cognac will work for you. Chances are they only worked for Dietrich and Roosevelt because they expected results. But, what you imbibe at night will certainly make some difference. We will now discuss those foods and drinks that have been known to influence sleep. We advise you to try those that appeal to you. Your final choice of snacks and nightcaps will be based on what works for you. If you find something promising, do it—even if it is eccentric.

In our chapter on food, we indicated that sugar, starch, salt, and caffeine affect sleep adversely. Obviously, if you cannot eliminate these items entirely, you should at least cut down, and restrict their intake to the earlier part of the day. You should also be careful of fruits at night if yours is a sleep onset problem. While great for your health, eating fruit at night may raise your blood sugar high enough to interfere with sleep.

Try to emphasize protein, calcium, and vitamin B foods in the evening. Keep your evening meal moderate, since overeating can destroy sleep. On the other hand, so can hunger. So find a sensible, happy medium that is right for you. Eat easily digested foods at night, and aim for getting to bed with a comfortable stomach—neither too full nor too empty.

For your snacks, dairy products may be best—they are rich in both protein and calcium, and usually high in l-tryptophan. If you are inclined to junkier kinds of snacks, try unsalted nuts or sunflower seeds.

Various cultures throughout the world have discovered their own effective sleep-inducing foods and beverages. Here are some of those that are viewed as credible:

• The Burmese eat pollen cakes at night. Pueblo Indians eat large amounts of mushrooms (which have a high content of B vitamins) right before bed. An ancient Chinese prescription for insomnia is to take an extract of chopped ginseng and dried orange peel, fortified with honey. It is to be drunk right before going to sleep. Interestingly, one of the active components of genseng is *saponin*, which has been used by Western doctors to treat hypertension and high blood pressure. (While ginseng is said to have marvelous curative powers, its use as a soporific has received mixed reviews. Said an angry friend to whom we recommended it, "Thanks, pal, I buzzed around the whole night as if I'd drunk ten cups of coffee.")

• An old English favorite is to eat a large apple, chewing it slowly, before going to bed. English farmers shared the following recipe for lettuce tea with the Romany Gypsies: Take the outside leaves of a large head of lettuce and put them in a saucepan with half a pint of boiling water. Add salt and simmer for 20 minutes. Strain and serve.

• The gypsies who have to deal with sleep problems caused by their constantly changing environments, also make an effective fruit drink that they take just before bed. Mix together the juice of one lemon and one orange in a glass with two tablespoons of honey. Fill the glass with hot water and drink slowly. Hot grapefruit juice is also used.

• From the countryside of Scotland comes this unappealing remedy for insomnia—oatmeal gruel. Fortunately, it is recommended with lots of honey. Closer to home is this remedy, sworn by among the well-rested farmers of Vermont: mix three tablespoons of apple cider vinegar with a cupful of honey. At bedtime, swallow two teasponfuls. If still awake in an hour, take two more teaspoonfuls, and keep doing that until you fall asleep.

• Two others that seem unappetizing, but come to us supported by considerable folk wisdom are, raw onions and olive oil. No, not together. The raw onions can be eaten on a slice of toast at bedtime. The olive oil should be taken after the evening meal and before bed—one teaspoon each time. An attractive way to do this, and one which insures easy digestion, is known as "orzone." Fill two dessertspoons with malted milk powder and pour them into a Horlick's mixer with one dessertspoon of olive oil. Add hot water and shake. Drink this no less than an hour before bedtime, since it is a rather concentrated food drink.

• The hardy Balkan mountaineers have an old tradition of drinking a glass of buttermilk a half-hour before bed. With this we come to soporifics that may carry with them a firm basis in scientific fact. Buttermilk is known to be an excellent source of calcium, which, as we saw in a previous chapter, is essential for proper sleep.

• Then there is the perennial hot milk. You will recall in our discussion of l-tryptophan that researchers now think the sleep-inducing effects of warm milk are attributable to the abundance of that amino acid. That and the calcium make hot milk a double threat for insomniacs. Heating it up also adds to its effect, for the warmth increases the flow of blood to the abdominal area, reducing the amount of blood in the head. Reduction of blood in the head is associated with restful sleep and it aids digestion.

Don't drink it too hot. If you like, add a teaspoon of honey, or malt powder. Postum or Ovaltine with the warm milk is also said to be beneficial.

Gaylord Hauser recommends his "sleep cocktail," a cup of hot milk with two teaspoons of the darkest molasses you can find. The B vitamins in the molasses add to the sedative effect.

Those with low blood sugar should find the milk drinks especially useful. Cheese or yogurt can be substituted for variety or preference. Remember to keep some protein food handy in case you wake up restless in the night.

• Along with your nightcap, you might want to take the following supplements: 10 milligrams of B_6; 100 milligrams of pantothenic acid; 250 milligrams of magnesium oxide; 500

milligrams of calcium lactate. A tablespoon of brewer's yeast added to your milk will do nothing for your taste buds, but it might help your sleep a good deal.

- Among the best nightcaps known for sleep are herbal teas, or *tisanes* as they are known in France.

Herbal Remedies for The Sleepless

The Ayur Veda, an Indian encyclopedia-scripture on the healing arts, was said to have been composed thousands of years ago when an ancient seer was walking in the forest and all the wild herbs sang to him of their curative powers. Around 3000 B.C. in China, the Emperor Shen Ung sang the glories of several hundred medicinal herbs. The clay tablets of ancient Sumerians and Assyrians, 4500 years old, record the attributes of some 250 herbs. In our own ancient roots, Hippocrates, the father of medicine, taught the value of herbs and extolled them as a possible panacea. Aristotle classified hundreds of herbs according to their specific effects.

Despite their illustrious past, herbs are the subject of some controversy among modern practitioners of medicine. Many feel that herbs have not been sufficiently tested and may contain harmful ingredients. The argument is countered by those who say that herbs are harmless and have been used effectively for far longer than modern drugs, whose safety is dubious.

Herbalists, who are not permitted to prescribe remedies because they are not licensed to practice medicine, have nonetheless put in print the known uses of herbs. Many are said to have an effective sedative and tranquilizing action without causing any side effects. Many of the herbs can be purchased at health food stores. The more exotic ones can be purchased from herbal supply houses listed in the Appendix. Most of the herbs recommended for insomnia are inexpensive, usually 50 cents to a dollar an ounce. Most of them can be grown in your own garden. If you care to try it, consult *The Herb Book* (Emmaus, PA: Rodale Press, 1972).

Here are the herbs known to be effective for encouraging sleep:

- The natives of the West Indies use *Passion Flower* tea before retiring.

• The Hopi Indians of the American southwest use several herbs to bring on sleep, the most effective being *Sand Verbena*. This tall, straggling herb with papery fruits, grows in abundance in the southwestern mesas. The Hopi use it particularly for helping their children sleep.

• *Catnip* is said to be an effective sedative that will quickly bring on drowsiness and a natural, deep sleep. We had a first hand verification of this recently, when a friend of ours was shaken up in a minor automobile accident. She was unable to settle down, and so we served her a cup of catnip tea. A half hour later she felt too sleepy to drive home. She awakened the next morning on our living room sofa, and said she slept more peacefully than she had in weeks.

• *Lime Blossom* tea is recommended as a harmless, pleasant bedtime drink, because the mineral traces it contains are said to be soothing to the nervous system. To add to its effectiveness a pinch of *Skullcap*—no more than can fit on a penny—can be mixed in.

• A nice combination drink that many have found helpful is the following: a spoonful each of *Valerian, Catnip, Skullcap,* and *Hops* in a pint of boiling water. Let it steep 15 minutes, and drink shortly before bedtime.

• *Primrose* tea is recommended for hypersensitive people, and for those who are high-strung and restless in bed.

• For general nervousness, *Rhododendron,* or "snow-rose," is suggested.

• For those who have nightmares, *Peony* and *Spurge Laurel* have been recommended.

• For twitching muscles, as well as dizziness and headaches that interfere with sleep, the choice seems to be *Hops.* Hops, by the way, is said to be rich in vitamin B, an excuse for much ale drinking in England. And pillows stuffed with hops are a commonly used folk remedy for insomnia. Warning: the smell of hops is rather powerful.

The granddaddy of all sleep-inducing herbs is *Chamomile.* This sweet, fragrant flower has been used for centuries as a safe, strong sedative. It is easy to obtain, even in tea bag form, at just about any health food store.

Chamomile's sedative effects recently had an unexpected verification from a team of scientists. The team, led by Dr. Lawrence Gould, was running a series of tests to see if chamomile had any effects on the cardiac conditions of patients who had undergone ventricular catheterizations. It had none. But the team was astonished to find a different reaction. Writing in the *Journal of Clinical Pharmacology* (January 10, 1974), Dr. Gould wrote: "A striking hypnotic [sleep-inducing] action of the tea was noted in ten of 12 patients. It is most unusual for patients undergoing cardiac catheterizations to fall asleep. The anxiety produced by this procedure as well as the pain associated with cardiac catheterizations all but preclude sleep. Thus, the fact that ten out of 12 patients fell into a deep slumber shortly after drinking camomile tea is all the more striking. Further investigations of the role of camomile tea as a hypnotic are therefore warranted."

There are many other herbs that are recommended for inducing sleep. We suggest the following books for general information: *Medical Botany*, by Lewis and Elvin-Lewis; *Mastering Herbalism*, by Paul Huson; *Herbs and Things*, by Jeanne Rose; *Herbs to Put You to Sleep*, by Ceres; and the popular *Back to Eden*, by Jethro Kloss. Another source of information is an herbal chart with cross-referenced herbs and ailments, by Leslie J. Kaslof.

Store your herbs in glass jars to keep out moisture, and keep them away from sunlight. Label your jars—many of the herbs look very much alike.

Wine

"Wine," said Benjamin Franklin, "is constant proof that God loves us and loves to see us happy."

For the insomniac, wine may, indeed, be a godsend at times. Earlier in the book, we stated that alcohol interferes with natural sleep when taken in immoderate amounts. However, for the person who feels the need for a stronger sleep-inducer than the mild ones we have discussed here (and that can occur on occasion to any of us), some wine is a reasonably safe sedative, and certainly preferable to drugs.

"Alcohol puts the higher brain center to sleep," says Dr. Joseph Mendels, director of the sleep laboratory at Philadelphia's VA Hospital. "It is a very good sedative, and many people will take a small tot of something before they go to bed; and while one doesn't want to recommend this as a routine for everybody, it may be less pernicious than some of the sleeping medications people take."

Because wine is absorbed slowly through the stomach, it produces a sustained and gentle tranquilizing effect. In scientific experiments conducted at the University of California School of Medicine, moderate doses of red wine were found to significantly lessen emotional tension.

Dr. Salvatore Lucia, an expert on the medicinal uses of wine, and author of *Wine and Your Well-Being*, says that a four-ounce serving of wine (about half a glass) taken on an empty stomach, or eight ounces taken with food, will produce a mildly tranquilized state. Taken half an hour to an hour before bedtime, a small glass of wine, says the doctor, will help produce drowsiness.

Apparently, wine is not the only alcoholic beverage recommended for sleep. Dr. Frederic Damrau studied 56 otherwise healthy middle-aged and elderly persons who had difficulty sleeping. The subjects were given an eleven-ounce bottle of stout to drink before retiring—one sixth the amount required to produce intoxication. Sleep improved in 76 percent of the cases. Dr. Damrau concludes: "Stout apparently has a large field of application as a relaxing agent for the average person who has ordinary difficulties with sleeping. Its use in preference to sleeping pills obviates the danger of drug addiction and other untoward effects."

Hops, by the way, the main ingredient in ale, is known to have a lot of B-vitamins.

Before you dash to the liquor store, however, keep in mind that these nightcaps should be used on a limited basis. Alcohol raises the sugar level, for one thing, which makes it inadvisable for diabetics and hypoglycemics, or for anyone who has found that sugar adversely affects sleep. Also, keep in mind that larger doses of alcohol can actually trigger the same response as a stimulant—the body will mobilize itself to prevent poisoning.

Cheers! And sweet dreams.

Your Bedroom Environment

Upon seeing a newspaper ad for 600 sleep-aid products, the irrepressible Ogden Nash wrote a poem cataloging the slumber buzzer, the eyeshade, the snore ball and the electric slippers, asking how come our ancestors were able to sleep so well without them? His point was well taken—there really should be no need for all the various gadgets that have been invented for insomniacs. We should be able to fall asleep under any circumstances, just as our hardy ancestors did. But they lived closer to nature, and they did not have to put up with annoyances like traffic noise and street lights. We have a penchant for devices, and the more elaborate the better. Everyone likes a new toy.

But often we rely on gadgets so we don't have to rely on ourselves. Remember, therefore, as we discuss the accoutrements of the optimal environment for sleep, that *you*, ultimately, are your best weapon against insomnia. Your goal should be self-sufficiency. That is, your mind and body should be so well tuned that you are able to fall asleep just about anywhere and under any circumstances, when you are tired. Nonetheless, the environment does, of course, make a difference, and should be considered an integral part of a holistic attack on sleep problems.

For our information on the sleeper's environment, we called on many sources, primarily the man who *Reader's Digest* says "cares more for your sleep than anyone else in the world." He is America's Public Sandman, Norman Dine.

Forty years ago Mr. Dine sold his furniture business in Massachussetts and set out to learn all he could about sleep and insomnia. He had been racked with sleeplessness for several years, had been to a battery of doctors whose standard advice was "don't worry." That was not enough for a man determined to join Nabokov's "moronic fraternity," and so he enrolled at Columbia Teachers College and studied mental hygiene. Later, he went to Chicago, and studied with the late Dr. Edmond Jacobson at his relaxation laboratory. He also studied the works of Dr. H. M. Johnson at Carnegie Tech, who was at that time one of the few people engaged in research on sleep.

Mr. Dine eventually got his own insomnia under control. It then occurred to him that he was an expert on the subject. He decided to combine that expertise with his knowledge of the furniture business. Thus, Norman Dine became America's first bona fide sleep merchant. His shop in New York became a haven for insomniacs, and the prototype for many imitations around the country.

Now around 70, give or take a few years, Mr. Dine holds forth at 33 Halsted Street in East Orange, New Jersey, just a short nap from New York. We visited him there and found him remarkably agile (we had difficulty keeping up with him as he led us around) and refreshingly congenial.

Mr. Dine divides human beings into two categories: the "constitutionally fortunate," and "light sleepers." The former do not need sleep shops. The others, the readers of this book presumably, are those of us who react unfavorably to irritations such as noise, light, pressure, heat, cold, drafts, stuffiness, humidity, caffeine, a restless spouse, and others. It is people in that category whose needs Norman Dine and his staff feel confident they can meet. He takes a four-pronged approach to subduing what he calls "the marathon mind"—sounds and rhythms, electric massage, aquatherapy, and techniques like Jacobson's, yoga, and TM to release tension. In addition, he provides learned counsel on mattresses, pillows, and other accessories, many of which he himself has invented, or designs and makes to order.

In the following pages we discuss various aspects of the bedroom environment, and describe the appropriate accessories as we go along.

Noise:

When Amy Lowell, the poet, stayed in a hotel, she would rent five rooms—one to sleep in and empty rooms on each side, above, and below. She couldn't tolerate noise.

Sleep specialists would probably say that Ms. Lowell heard the noise because she was a poor sleeper, not vice versa. Nonetheless, noise can be a bother.

Mankind has long known the effects of sounds, both good and bad. We know, for example, that certain sounds have a soothing, lulling, restful effect. Those are the sounds that we choose when we want to listen to relaxing music, for example. We have created lullabies to guide our babies gently into sleep. For that purpose, a Sousa march will not do. We seek the quiet sounds of the woods, or the somnolent sound of waves lapping a shore, when we need repose.

When we need to stir the mind and soul to action we use rousing drumbeats and trumpets. And when we want to drive our fellow creatures out of their minds, we use harsh, jarring, dissonant sounds. Sometimes we do it involuntarily, as in the case of a factory in France where workers suddenly complained of nausea, fatigue, and irritability for no apparent reason. It was discovered later that a new set of machines had been installed, and the sounds they produced were, although beyond the range of human hearing, upsetting the nervous systems of the workers.

The autonomic nervous system, which controls involuntary activities like heart beat, begins to react to sounds at 70 decibels. Sounds above that threshold, especially those that are irregular, unpredictable, and meaningless, raise the diastolic blood pressure, and cut down the supply of blood to the heart. As the intensity increases, the emergencylike response gets more severe: pupils dilate; mouth and tongue get dry; leg, abdomen, and chest muscles contract; heartbeat quickens, and adrenalin pours forth. There is some indication that exposure to high volume noise raises the likelihood of heart attacks.

Here is a sampling of the decibel counts of some common noisemakers: a jet plane on takeoff-150 (120 is the pain threshold); a riveter-130; a group of electric guitars-114; a loud power motor-107; an outboard motor-102; a pneumatic jackhammer-94; a blender-93; a sports car or truck-90; a vacuum cleaner-81.

Unfortunately, those are sounds that are often in the air when people are asleep. Saddest of all, the sound of traffic on a relatively quiet city street is approximately 70 decibels, just about the level at which the autonomic nervous system begins to respond. And it responds even when we are asleep. Even if the sounds do not wake you, or prevent you from falling asleep, the slight arousal that they elicit will prevent you from getting the most beneficial sleep.

What to do?

Move to the countryside, for one thing. But that is not always convenient. Nor is it always quiet. Superhighways and teenagers with electric rock guitars are everywhere.

One solution is to use earplugs. There are several good types on the market. The cheap kind designed to keep water out of the ears of swimmers is not recommended for noise. A product called Ear Defender, manufactured by Mine Safety Appliances Company of Pittsburgh, is made of soft, rubbery plastic, preshaped to fit the ear opening properly. They come in three sizes—small, medium, and large. Since you can get a pair for about a dollar, we recommend you buy one of each to test for size.

Flents Inc. of Norwalk, Connecticut, makes a wax earplug that is quite effective. Soft and malleable, the plugs can be rolled into a ball, inserted in the ear opening without having to be pressed too deeply toward the ear drum, and molded to cover the outer part of the ear opening. Quite good at muffling even the sound of heavy traffic, the plugs come in small boxes of four pairs for two dollars. Their big disadvantage is that the wax rubs off. This means buying a new box every so often depending on how much you use them. We known someone who uses them five nights a week—it's quiet on weekends—and goes through a box every two to three months. It also means that some of the wax rubs off in your ear. While that appears to be easily countered by soap and water, we do not know what effects there might be if the wax happened to drip into the ear opening.

Our personal favorite is the E-A-R Plugs, by the E-A-R Corporation. Made of a form of polymer, an "exclusive energy-absorbing material," the plugs feature a time-delayed expansion. Rolled into a narrow cylinder and inserted in the ear, the plug expands to a virtually unnoticed, but snug fit that conforms to the shape of almost any normal ear canal.

E-A-R plugs cost $1.50 a pair, or $14.00 for a dozen pair—they do wear thin after some time—and can be ordered from Time and Space Enterprises, 650 N. Bronson Lane, Hollywood CA. 90004.

But earplugs cannot eliminate all noise, although they will certainly muffle anything that comes along. Moreover, some people do not like complete silence, preferring sleep-conducive sounds instead. What do you do if gentle raindrops, soothing wind, or rolling surf is unavailable when you want to sleep? You can buy an electronic Sleep Coaxer for one thing. This handy device weighs only two pounds and is only seven inches wide. It masks out disturbing sounds with drowsing sounds of surf, rain, or wind. Complete with a volume control, the machine costs $90. A less expensive model, which has the sound of rain and a plain, "white" sound, costs $65.

Also available is Marpac Company's Sleep-Mate, which creates an adjustable, windlike sound. Compact and portable, the device has been tested at a major sleep laboratory and found to be harmless, and not to interfere with normal sleep cycles. It is said to have a lulling effect that might be useful even for insomniacs who are not bothered by noise. Like the Sleep Coaxer already mentioned, it is designed for continuous operation and consumes no more electricity than a small night light. Cost: $25.

That certain sounds can help you sleep has been verified by hundreds of stories of people who can't get to sleep without their favorites, like a roaring stream that might keep a city person awake, or the ticking of a grandfather clock. Most of us know people who fall asleep with the TV or radio on, only to wake with a start when someone shuts it off. Scientists have found that newborn infants can be lulled to sleep with recordings of simulated versions of their mother's heartbeat.

The advantage of the mechanical sound conditioners is that, in most cases, they have been carefully constructed to produce a bland, low-frequency sound that blends with other sounds present and can modify even sharp and unexpected sounds, thus reducing the severity of their impact. The extremes are less extreme, and therefore less annoying.

A breaking-in period may be required. A friend almost smashed his because he was so annoyed by the device. He stuck it out though, and soon became used to it. He says that from that point on he slept better than ever.

If you have trouble breaking in your sound conditioner, start by using it for a short period of time before going to bed. Increase the time gradually, and also increase the volume. Soon, the sound will become part of the background and you will forget that it is present.

Many people think that friendly noises are useless unless they block out other sounds completely. This is not so. To do that, the sound would have to be louder than the loudest harmful sound, and would then be harmful itself. The intention is simply to mask existing sounds.

Your fan, or the buzz of your air conditioner might do the job for you. But when you don't want the cooling, try the devices we mentioned. Or, alternatively, create your own device by taping the sounds that suit your needs. Make sure you get a recorder that shuts off by itself (the disadvantage here is that you don't get the sound through the night, but you may only need it to fall asleep).

In the eighteenth century, a young prince suffering from a severe case of insomnia asked his protegé, a young musician named Goldberg, to help him with his sleep problem. Goldberg took the request to his teacher, who composed a slow, enchanting piece of piano music for the prince. The composer was Johann Sebastian Bach, and the piece of music came to be known as the *Goldberg Variations*. It worked for the prince and you will find it very soothing too, particularly in recordings of solo piano.

We called a few musicians and music teachers, asking them to recommend music-to-fall-asleep-by. The variation of responses was astonishing. The only common factor was—classical music is best, and nonsymphonic music is more likely to be quiet and lyrical enough not to stir the senses. As a result of our poll, we can state unequivocally that it all depends on your taste and mood.

Music that was most often mentioned: Brahm's *Lullaby*; Schubert's *Serenade*; Debussy's *Afternoon of a Faun,* and *Girl With Flaxen Hair*; Wagner's *Siegfried Idyll*; Beethoven's *Pastoral Symphony* (beware of the storm sequence); Mozart quartets; Chopin nocturnes; and chamber music by Bach, Schumann, and any composer of your liking. Guitar and harp music were given general approval.

Darkness:

We have all had the experience of trying to darken our minds for sleep in a bedroom with too much light. Light is stimulating. It is said that more than 80 percent of all sensory information comes to us in the form of light through our eyes. A British scientist once studied the stimulating effects of light by measuring the activity of the kidneys. It went down significantly in a darkened room. Closing your eyes is not enough. Some light comes through.

A fine eyeshade called simply the Sleep Shade, is manufactured by a company in San Francisco, and it comes in plain black sateen at $4.25.

We have found the shade to be effective in keeping out all light rays. It may take a night or two to get used to having it on; you might be very conscious of it at first. But, soon enough, it becomes a part of your milieu. It can be worn fairly loose without reducing effectiveness, and it has a soft, stuffed pad for the bridge of the nose.

But what if you are afraid of the dark or can't sleep in a completely dark room? If you require *some* light, make it soft, and indirect. You can buy the claustrophobic's eyeshade. Its tiny pinholes let some light in, but keep the light subdued.

Those of you who like a dark room but sleep with a spouse who stays up later to read, might consider the Spot Lamp that clamps onto your headboard and projects a clear, nonglare beam. According to the brochure, it "leaves you in soothing darkness and lets him finish the chapter."

Your Bed

O bed! O bed! Delicious bed!
That heaven on earth to the weary head!
—Thomas Hood

We spend over one-third of our lives in bed, so we owe it to ourselves to have the right kind of bed. Just what "right" is varies with each individual. Queen Esther, the first person in the Bible whose bed is mentioned, slept on a bunch of cushions flung into a corner. Nero's bed was a little more ornate, encrusted with precious stones alleged to have beneficial powers—rubies, amethysts, garnets, and diamonds. King Louis XIV of France owned 413 beds. And Benjamin Franklin, a fanatic for cool-air sleeping, kept four in his room so that he could rotate as each became warm.

Perhaps the first bed question we should address is the delicate one of single vs. double beds. Among married insomniacs the issue frequently comes up in the offices of marriage counselors. We recommend twin beds. Dr. P. J. Steincrohn says, "There is more likelihood of loss of sleep and consequent irritability and argument in double beds than in twin beds (no elbows in the ribs, no twisting and turning)."

If, as a couple, your preferences for bedroom conditions are irreconcilable, you might consider sleeping in separate rooms, or at least be prepared for that contingency at times when it is needed. The same is true in the event of snoring, about which more later on. It might seem unromantic to split up the marriage bed that way, but better the bed than the marriage. We are never more irrational, nor more pugnacious, than when we are tired and someone else—no matter how dear—disturbs our sleep.

If you do choose mutual exile, don't fret. Make the best of it. Think how romantic a surprise visit can be.

Your Mattress: Most back specialists advocate the use of a firm mattress. Dr. Leon Root, an orthopedist and coauthor of *Oh, My Aching Back,* says that a hard foam mattress, four to six inches thick on a platform foundation, or a one-inch thick plywood board, is the best thing for an aching back. Firm mattresses, he says, "tend to keep the lower back from sagging."

We have all been conditioned by advertisers to want a firm mattress, and if Dr. Root is correct, we probably should—if we have bad backs. But, according to Norman Dine, many people are sleeping on mattresses that are actually *too* firm for their own good. He emphasizes fitting your mattress to your individual needs. Over his long years as a sleep consultant, he has evolved a way of determining the right degree of firmness for each individual. Such factors as height, weight, shape, posture, sleep pattern, and sensitivity variables like irritability to pressure, excessive curvature of the back, weak or long back, are all considered.

His golden rule seems to be, the light sleeper should avoid as many irritants as possible. For example, your mattress should be eight to ten inches longer than your height, and seven to ten inches wider than you are. If you *literally* slept like a log—that is, if you didn't move—then that would not be necessary. But, even the most loglike sleepers change position about 20 times in a night, and some of us change 50 or more times. We need room to move comfortably.

The moving about also changes the parts of the body that are subject to pressure, and it redistributes circulation flow. If your bed is too soft or too hard, your *motility* (spontaneous movements) will be restricted.

Here are some rules by which you can evaluate your mattress:

If there is painful pressure at the heavier parts of your body such as the hips, if your positions seem insecure, and if the number of different positions you can assume comfortably is limited, and if there is coolness under your body, then your mattress is probably *too firm*. Thin people, by the way, whose bones are not well cushioned, usually need more resiliency and less firmness, for a hard mattress will press excessively against parts of the body. If you have a curvature of the back, a hard mattress will probably be painful.

If you have back fatigue, a sagging spine, if you feel undue body warmth in bed, if you feel a swaying sensation and restricted movement, chances are your mattress is *too soft*.

What you should look for is effortless bouyancy, a cradling sensation, even support, complete freedom of movement, and gentle pressure evenly distributed over your whole body. Says Dr. W. W. Bauer, "The best condition for good sleep is gentle support of the body at all points, without too much pressure at the shoulder or hips, and without permitting too much lateral bending of the spine."

When mattress shopping, always lie down on the mattress; don't just push and prod. Stretch out and relax on it. Hunt around. Find one that feels just right, keeping in mind such factors as bouyancy, resiliance, and silence (no squeaking springs). Look for lots of quilting. Don't be carried away by pretty designs. Inspect the warranty—federal regulations state that it must spell out all details in plain language—and look for a long warranty. Look for a mattress with a coil count of at least 300 for every 54 inches of mattress in an inner spring unit. Remember that while a smooth surface may look more aesthetic, the tufted mattress is better and will retain its shape and nonsagging quality much longer. Check beyond the name of the model; manufacturers often call identical mattresses by different names so they can be sold at different prices.

Once you purchase a mattress, treat it well, so that it will give you maximum service over time. Break it in correctly. During the first six months of use, turn it over once a month, and turn it end-to-end at the same time. After that, do it twice a year. Once a month air it out with the windows open, and vacuum it thoroughly—even the box spring. Always use a mattress pad.

Another factor to keep in mind is allergies. Many people are allergic to the kapok used to stuff some mattresses. Others are allergic to foam, horsehair, or feathers. Such allergies, says Dr. Claude A. Frazier, afflict 15 to 20 percent of us. If you find yourself coughing or wheezing at night, if you have headaches or snore excessively, and if you have dark circles under your eyes even when rested, you might be allergic to your mattress. Dr. Frazier recommends rigorous vacuuming of mattresses to keep out the dust, which is a common irritant. Avoid tufted mattresses if you have allergic symptoms. Use well-washed bedclothes. Wrap everything in protective covers, which you can obtain from Allergen Proof Encasings, 3 Park Place, New York, N.Y., 10007. Tape up the zippers.

Your pillow: The Japanese rest their heads on blocks of wood. The Zulus also sleep on wood, delicately carved. In Czarist Russia, children were given elegant little pillows, trimmed with lace, called *doumkas*—"the one you tell your thoughts to."

Pillows should be just thick enough to hold the head in the same relation to the shoulders and spine that it has when standing up. One way to test it out is to stand sideways against a wall with your shoulder touching the wall. Place the pillow on your shoulder. It should fit perfectly between your head and the wall.

If your pillow is too thick, it can strain the neck muscles. If your head sinks too deeply into the pillow, it could cause overheating and make a change of position more difficult. In addition, the strain on the shoulder muscles from a wrongly positioned pillow can cut off circulation to the arms and hands, causing a "pins and needles" sensation that will probably wake you up. There is no scientific evidence to support the theories that raising the head to drain blood from it, or lowering the head to increase blood flow to the brain— both of which have been lauded as beneficial—have any validity.

Goose down pillows are lusciously comfortable, and with proper care will last 25 years or more. Since down is very expensive, most feather pillows also include duck, chicken, and turkey feathers. These also provide extra body.

Most pillows nowadays are made of synthetic materials, which are better for allergy sufferers. The best is said to be "continuous multifilament fiber." It is spun into the casing, and comes in a wide range of different degrees of firmness. It does not shift, settle, or wad up. Most synthetics last for five to seven years, and cost about $10 to $15.

The trouble with most pillows is that they do not respect the contours of the body. Someone made them box-shaped, and box-shaped they remained. Dine's has designed a contour pillow that elevates the head without irritating the shoulders. It is crescent shaped, permitting the head to rest tranquilly without the pillow's bunching up.

Most experts say that sleeping on your side in the manner described in the next chapter is ideal, However, it takes a long time for anyone to learn new sleep positions, and we will shift back into undesirable positions in our sleep. Sleeping on the back is not recommended, but for those who do, there is Dr. Jackson's Neck Pillow. Cylindrical, and filled with a soft, malleable filling, it self-adjusts to the contours of your neck, cradling it and protecting the neck muscles, which can get seriously damaged from sleeping on your back incorrectly.

Sleep shops also have a variety of pillows for special purposes: some for raising either the head or the feet for those with particular breathing or circulation problems; and foam bolster pillows in different wedgelike shapes for sitting up and reading, or for placing under your knees (many people find their circulation greatly aided by having their knees elevated).

Blankets and sheets: There is no end to the variety of sheets and blankets now available. They come in all conceivable materials and colors. As for sheets, silk is the preferred choice, of course, if you can afford it. Cotton is perhaps next best because its natural texture will create less discomfort and less of the static electricity that often comes from rubbing against synthetics, a factor which doctors are becoming concerned about. But for the most part, you should select material that feels comfortable, and which does not offend any allergies you may have.

As for color, you have a wide choice. One manufacturer suggests pastels or neutral colors, such as beige, for those whose days are hectic; and deep, bold colors for those whose days are dull.

Louis Cheskin of the Color Research Institute of America, has discovered some fascinating effects of color that are of special interest to those with sleep problems. While subtle, and largely unconscious, the effects of colors can be profound. Red, he points out, has a violently stimulating effect, while blue, the coldest of all colors, is a sedative.

Blue has been used to calm, subdue, and soothe mental agitation. A Scandinavian physicist named Oscar Brunler suggested that all poor sleepers should use pale blue sheets, and sleep in blue pajamas. "If you are a poor sleeper," he wrote, "visualize blue all around you."

The greens are said to be good too. It is well known that green is the most soothing light vibration, one reason, perhaps, why the lush green of the countryside makes us feel so good.

These factors may seem trivial, and probably they are, but if you are not sleeping well, you can use all the help you can get. So why not consider a color change for sheets, and maybe even for wallpaper, paint, or pajamas as well?

Of course the basic thing about sheets is that they must be clean, smooth, and cool. The top sheet should be fitted rather loosely at the foot—for some reason, we tend to make our beds in such a way that our feet are inhibited. They should have room to maneuver, lest they get cramped and wake us up.

Blankets are a less trivial concern. A study by General Electric revealed that differences as small as one degree higher or lower in bed temperature made a noticeable difference in the quality of sleep. How heavily a sleeper should be blanketed is an individual matter, having to do largely with the discharge of body heat. Those of us who lose more heat than others need heavier covering than others who hold sufficient heat on their own.

Ideally, an electric blanket should be thermostatically controlled to respond to the temperature of the body as it changes. Such a blanket was actually produced and it worked perfectly—in the laboratory. For some reason, it never worked in the hands of consumers. It was too delicate, they say. So, electric blankets with thermostatic controls respond to the temperature of the room, not the body. Good, but not ideal.

Your blankets should not be too heavy. Consider this: in eight hours of sleep you lift your bedclothes at least 7,000 times by breathing. In addition to electric blankets, eiderdown comforters, and various kinds of quilts, can provide excellent insulation without weighing you down. Experiment to find the best for you.

The choice is wide ranging—several varieties of electrics, and different wools and acrylics. You can even buy an automatic bed warmer that fits between the mattress and the sheets to provide warmth from beneath you in winter.

Temperature and the air you breathe: During your sleep, you breathe in over 25 barrels of air. Why not have it be the best?

Ben Franklin lived to be 84 years old at a time when the life expectancy was only 35. Perhaps one reason was his ability to sleep soundly. Here is his prescription:

> When you are waked up by uneasiness, and find you cannot sleep easily again, get out of bed, beat up and turn up your pillow, shake the bed clothes well with at least twenty shakes, then throw the bed open and leave it to cool; in the meanwhile, continuing undressed, walk about your chamber, till your skin has had time to discharge its load, which it will do sooner, as the air may be drier and colder.
>
> When you begin to feel the cold air unpleasant, then return to your bed; you will soon fall asleep, and your sleep will be sweet and pleasant.

It is hard to say whether it was the freshness of the air or its coolness that helped Mr. Franklin sleep. Both, however, are said to be important.

The best temperature for sound sleep is between 60 and 64 degrees F. Sleep researchers have found that people tend to need more sleep when the bedroom temperature is lower than 60°, and are less likely to sleep long enough to feel rested if the bedroom temperature is above 70° F. While the main concern is your individual comfort—which may well require a temperature outside the range mentioned above—most experts seem to lean toward cooler temperatures. One possible reason for this is that body temperature usually begins to fall as a person approaches bedtime, rising again before he awakens.

In cold weather, an electric blanket is often preferred. A blanket *under* the bottom sheet is an excellent idea.

Cold feet, which often keep us awake in winter, can usually be remedied by heavy socks. Charles Darwin rarely slept without them. If you need something more, sporting goods stores and camping supply houses sell a wide variety of light, unobtrusive feet warmers, made of goose down and other material. Or you can purchase an electric warming pad that goes under your sheet to keep your feet warm by thermostatic control.

Keeping the room warm without parching it can be done with the aid of a humidifier, ranging from a small portable for $30 to a large console for over $100.

In hot weather, air conditioning is useful, of course, although many people complain about the artificiality of the air and prefer to use a fan. It is said that a cool top sheet is better, even on the hottest nights, than no top sheet at all. It is also said that you should avoid the temptation of cooling off with a cold shower before bed. It will stimulate your body to produce more heat.

A traditional balm used by Jews in the Middle East is a cool compress applied to the head at bedtime. Hot, congested head and eyes are among the causes of sleeplessness. Bathe the eyes with cold water, and use a cold-water compress on the eyelids and forehead, before going to bed.

As for ventilation, there is some debate about that. While common sense and most experts argue against stuffy rooms, others point to the fact that it is in those very stuffy rooms that we tend to get drowsy. Watch what happens in a conference room in the winter when the windows are closed. The advocates of stuffy rooms say that if you air out the room before bed, take in a few deep breaths and have reasonably healthy lungs, you will have all the air you need, with plenty to spare. Dr. Charles Kelly, whose breathing method we shall describe in the next chapter, demonstrated that two sleeping people cannot use up enough air in an ordinary-sized bedroom for either to notice the difference.

Then there is the story of that classic fresh-air fiend, Ben Franklin, who once had to share a room with a man who could not sleep with the window open. As might be expected, Franklin won the ensuing debate, and the shutters were opened wide. Franklin slept perfectly, and the poor loser did not sleep a wink. But, in the morning, they discovered that the shutters they had opened onto the fresh night air actually opened onto a small closet. Is the answer to the ventilation debate, "it's all in the mind"?

Yoga and Other Exercises

The science of Yoga dates back thousands of years to its roots in ancient India. In the recent past much misconception has arisen in the West that has, unfortunately, turned some people who might have benefited from it away from Yoga. Fortunately, that situation is now being corrected. Even medical science recognizes many of the health-giving, life-supporting advantages of this ancient wisdom.

Still, there are self-styled Yoga "experts" who may lead you in the wrong direction, so be discriminating. Be especially leery of meditation techniques taught under the name of Yoga that involve any degree of mental control or concentration.

Having issued that warning, let us turn to the particular uses of Yoga that are of importance to sleep. One entire branch of Yoga—the one most of us are familiar with—specializes in physical exercises. Simple, nonstrenuous, and remarkably beneficial, these are usually done during the day. Many people do them routinely in the morning or afternoon and enjoy a boost of energy, and noticeable relaxation. You should consult a Yoga book, or take a Yoga class, to learn a full set of exercises for use during the day. They will surely help your sleep, because they have an overall normalizing effect on the nervous system, and on key organs and glands. If you practice TM, do the Yoga postures before meditation.

Here we shall show you how to do the few exercises that most authorities recommend for insomnia. Ordinarily a full set of exercises is not advised for use at night—they are energizing. Done correctly, however, the following will help you get rid of the stress and tension that interfere with sleep. Some of the exercises will bend and twist the spine, thus freeing the flow of energy. Others will loosen and relax various muscles and joints. They will also give a valuable internal massage to vital organs such as the heart, liver, kidneys, and stomach. Their soothing influence on the nervous system should help restore the natural biorhythmic functions of the body.

These exercises are especially good for people who have sedentary jobs. Physical inactivity can devitalize the body and render it sluggish. These postures will stimulate proper circulation and help remove the sort of free-floating anxiety that gnaws at you at bedtime.

Here are some general points to keep in mind when doing any of the exercises. First, the word "exercise" is probably ill-advised. They are called *asanas* in India, a word that means "posture." That implies something less strenuous than the word "exercise," and for good reason. Westerners are used to exercises like calisthenics that raise the metabolism and build muscles through exertion. They have their advantages, of course. But *asanas* are not exercises of that type. They are meant to conserve, not use, energy.

It is very important to do these *asanas* slowly, gently, and comfortably. *Never strain, and never force your body into any position that is painful.* The postures as illustrated will look impossible. For most of us, they probably are. You have, more than likely, never bent or twisted or stretched in the ways called for. *It does not matter whether or not you can achieve the position illustrated.* What matters is that you move, slowly and easily, in the direction of the final posture, and *stop when you begin to feel a strain.* Hold at that point, and consider it done. Gradually, and all by itself, the body will become more flexible. The important thing is doing the postures, not achieving them. Yoga is not a contest. Straining to bend an extra inch will get you nothing but a pulled muscle, and that will keep you awake.

The Cobra: This *asana* should promote relaxation, particularly in the upper back and neck. The muscles supporting the spine are stretched and firmed, and several important organs are given stimulation. This *asana* is especially popular among people who bend over a desk all day.

Lie with your arms at your sides with your forehead touching the floor. Slowly, tilt your head back. Using your back muscles, raise your trunk as far off the floor as possible without using your hands. Keep your eyes open, and pretend you are trying to see as far behind you as you can, lifting first your head, then your neck, shoulders, and back. Place your hands as illustrated, beneath the shoulders. The fingers may be pointed toward one another, or straight ahead. With the head tilted backward (careful not to strain the neck muscles) push up gently and slowly. You should feel the back stretch, almost one vertebra at a time. Remember, these are not pushups. Your arms should not be doing much work. They

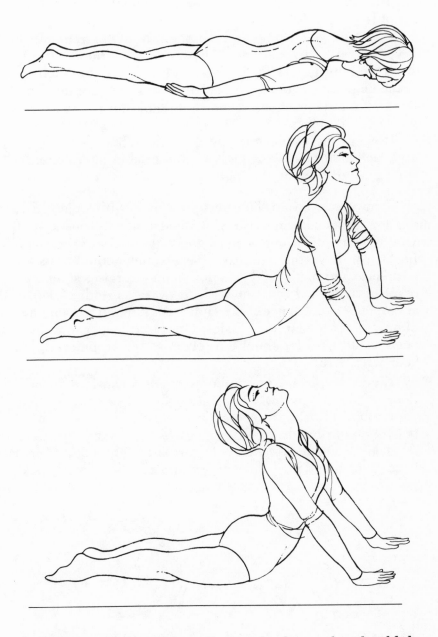

are there for support primarily; your back muscles should do most of the lifting.

Go up only as far as you can without strain. In the extreme position, the arms are straight and the head is tilted far back. The legs should be relaxed throughout, not tensed

195

up. Hold the position that you have comfortably attained for about ten seconds.

Keeping your spine arched, begin to lower yourself by reversing the procedure. The neck and head should straighten out last, with the forehead returning to touch the floor. Then bring your arms back to your sides, and turn your head so that your cheek rests comfortably on the floor. Let your body go limp.

Repeat the *asana* once again. Remember, do it slowly and easily, stop when it feels uncomfortable, and keep the back arched. Breathe normally throughout.

The Neck Twist: The neck area is easily subjected to tension, especially in those who are sedentary. Look around you at your office and see all the people contorting their necks to relieve the stiffness. Those spontaneous twists are imprecise and haphazard. The following exercises should be done in a relaxed manner with the eyes closed. Make no attempt to crack the neck with sudden or forceful movements. Simply turn as far as possible, stopping when straining begins, and hold for about ten seconds. As you proceed, the neck will gradually loosen.

Begin by placing your elbows on a level surface, like the floor, a table, or a desk. Your arms should be parallel, and your elbows fairly close together as you place your head between your hands.

Clasp your hands on the lower part of the back of your head. You should not be clasping your neck. Now gently push

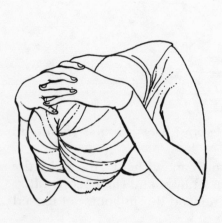
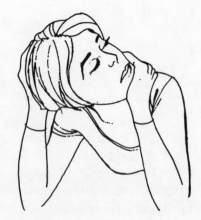

down until your chin touches your chest. Make sure that your elbows are close together, so that you have enough height to move your head downward. Hold for about ten seconds.

Without moving your arms, turn your head slowly and rest your chin in your left hand, so that the fingers rest on the *left* cheek. Grip the back of your head firmly with your right hand. Make sure your hands are gripping securely. Now turn your head slowly to the left, as far as possible. Hold for ten seconds, eyes closed.

Now, without moving the arms, turn your head slowly to the right and rest your chin in your right palm. This time the fingers should rest along the *right* cheek. Grip the back of your head with your left hand, firmly. Again, turn the head as far as possible, to the right this time. Slowly. Hold the extreme position for about ten seconds.

Remember in doing these neck twists that you want to turn the head as far as it will go. For this, you should use your hands, for doing so will give it just that extra twist which will make a big difference.

Do each of the three positions once.

Alternate Leg Pulls: Sit with your legs stretched out before you. Place the right heel firmly against the inside of your left thigh. Reach up, lean backward slightly, and then bend forward, taking a firm hold on your left leg or ankle, or, if you are particularly flexible, your foot. Now gently pull your trunk downward *without straining*. Your head limp, move in the direction of touching your forehead to your knee. More likely than not, you will feel a strain in the back of your outstretched leg, and in your back, long before your head is anywhere near your knee. Hold it right there. Eventually the leg and back muscles will stretch, and you will bend forward further. Be satisfied in the knowledge that you are getting as much out of the *asana* as you can—and that is considerable—by bending even slightly forward in this manner.

Hold at your point of maximum stretch for about 30 seconds, or as long as it is comfortable. Then repeat the *asana* with your right leg outstretched. Do it twice each way.

Remember when doing the leg pull that you should grasp your outstretched leg as far forward as is comfortable. For some, that might mean the toes or the middle of the foot.

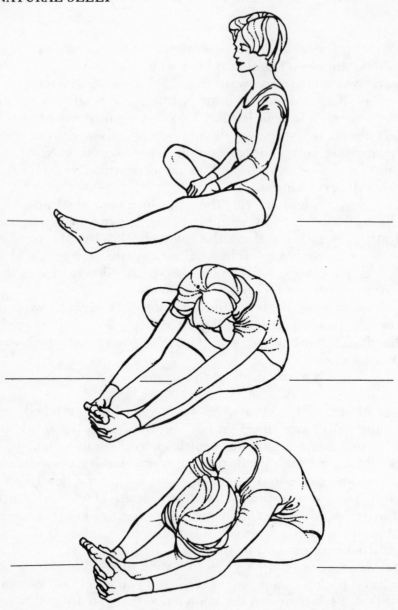

For others, less flexible, it might mean the knee. Also remember that the leg that is folded will have a tendency to lift up. This is natural, and will occur less frequently as you progress. Your outstretched knee might also lift up. If this happens, you have probably reached too far forward for your degree of flexibility. Grip the leg further up the body, thereby giving the back more of an opportunity to stretch. This *asana* is excellent for relieving tension in the legs, and aiding in leg circulation, a big factor in insomnia.

Shoulder Stand: The shoulder stand will have a noticeable effect on your blood circulation. You will feel a sensation of increased blood flow in the neck, throat and head. You will also feel a sensation of relaxation in the legs, as the pressure of the blood held down by the force of gravity is relieved. The posture rests the valves in the veins of the legs that keep blood flowing upward when we are upright. It allows a rich supply of blood to enter the regions above the heart, especially the brain, which is dependent on an adequate supply of blood. In many ways then, the shoulder stand can be of great value, *if you do it right.*

Lie flat with your arms at your sides. Brace the palms against the floor, stiffen your abdomen and leg muscles, and slowly raise your legs. When your legs are upright, perpendicular to your body, swing them back so that your hips leave the floor. Then prop your hands against your hips. Straighten up slowly. You may find it easiest to remain in a position with your hips only slightly off the floor, as in the third illustration. If you can, straighten up still further, but please do not be in any hurry to do so. You will get the most out of this *asana* by being conservative.

In the completed shoulder stand, the legs will be absolutely straight, and the chin will press against the chest. The body should not be rigid, it should be relaxed. *The weight should not be on your head or neck.* Having it there will damage the upper neck vertebrae. Your shoulders, upper back, and your supporting hands should bear the weight. You needn't hold your legs stiff. Flex or move them as comfortable. Hold for a maximum of half a minute.

Coming out is as important as going in to this posture. Be careful not to collapse out of it, crashing to the floor. Bend your knees and lower your legs. Place the hands by your side for support. Then roll forward slowly and carefully. When your buttocks touch the floor, hold there, straighten out your legs, and slowly lower them to the floor. Allow your body to go limp, and rest for a while.

If you find it too difficult to do the shoulder stand, a good alternative—and one you should be aware of even if you do

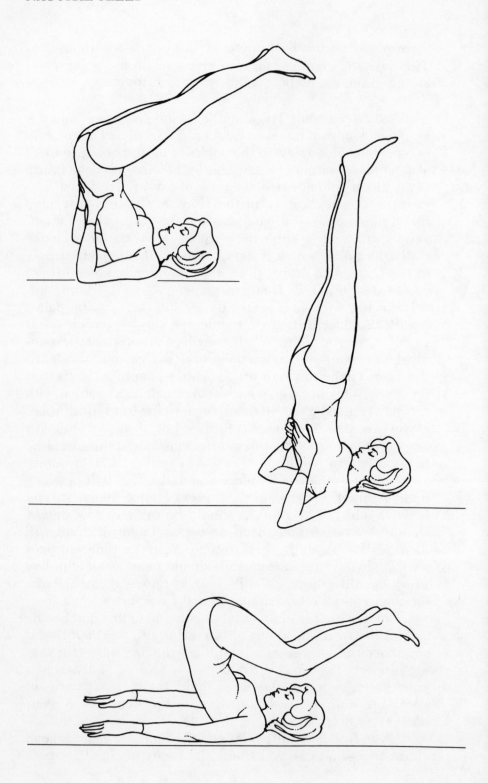

not do any of the Yoga exercises—is the use of a slant board.

Many sporting and specialty shops can supply you with one. They come with straps or bars to hook your feet under, and they generally fold up for easy storage. Some even come with built-in vibrators.

If you want to construct your own, all you need is a board the length of your body. Raise the foot of it 12 to 15 inches off the ground, and figure out some way to keep yourself from sliding down onto your head as you lie inverted.

Gaylord Hauser, the well-known health expert, calls this the "magic Yoga Slant," and urges his students to do it. Lying on the slant board for a few minutes before going to bed will be tremendously relaxing. It will also aid circulation considerably, and help bring the spine and certain inner organs into proper alignment. Hauser suggests you add a minute to your slanted time every few days until you can recline comfortably for 15 minutes.

Whether you use the slant board or the shoulder stand, you would do well to spend some time in a reversed position before bed.

The Corpse Pose: Despite its rather dismal name, this pose is everyone's favorite. You simply lie supine, hands at your side as illustrated, and relax completely. It is a perfect way to end your set of *asanas* in the evening, after coming down from the shoulder stand. Keep your palms up and your heels together. Relax.

Authorities differ on what you should do with your mind as you lie there. To some, the intention to relax, after having done the other *asanas*, should be sufficient to bring about the desired calmness. Others suggest deliberate relaxing of individual muscle groups. We will tell you how they recommend that be done, but we caution you against concentrating too hard. Your mind should be easy, not trying to force the body to relax. Straining will bring about the reverse of relaxation.

Those who advocate deliberate relaxation, suggest putting your attention first on the tips of your toes, then gradually up the leg—foot, ankle, calf, knee, thigh, etc. Some use the word *concentrate*; we chose not to, for it implies the sort of mind control that might be strenuous. Just let your attention fall easily where you are directing it, without attempting to drive away other thoughts, or to hold it rigidly in place. Be

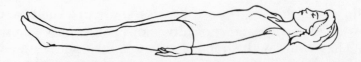

nonchalant. As you draw the attention to these areas, simply let them relax. Continue to draw your awareness up through the torso, neck, arms and face, lingering a while on each without rushing.

If done during the day following a complete set of *asanas*, the corpse pose should be done for only half a minute to a minute. Since you are doing it at night, with the intention of courting sleep, do it until you feel calm. However, don't overdo it, or you will end up fast asleep on your floor. Surely that is better than lying awake in bed, but not as good as slipping securely to slumber under the covers.

Some final points about doing these Yoga exercises: do them on a carpeted floor, with a good, thick blanket under you. It is especially important that the shoulder stand be done on a soft, well-cushioned surface.

Many of you may be familiar with the Head Stand, often shown in Yoga books, and may be tempted to do it instead of the shoulder stand. Don't! Unless done under the careful supervision of a Yoga master—not just a self-taught instructor—it can be dangerous. Too much pressure on the delicate blood vessels feeding the brain can be damaging.

Dress in loose clothing for your Yoga, and do it in a quiet, softly lit room. Since our concern is sleep, you might do them in your pajamas, beside your bed. Then you can slip right under the covers after you've done the corpse pose.

If you intend to eat or drink before retiring, do so *after* you have done the *asanas*, or wait sufficient time to digest. That might be 15 minutes or half an hour in the case of a drink or a light snack, or it might mean three or four hours in the case of a full meal.

And remember, never strain. Slow and easy does it.

Other exercises: We discussed Yoga in this section and aerobics earlier because your evening routine should be slow and easy. We even limited the Yoga postures to those recommended for bedtime—others might stir up energy. There are, however, other forms of exercise that, while perhaps not as beneficial to overall health as Yoga, are good to do before sleep to take the edge off, and to smooth out a possibly sluggish circulation.

Dancing is a good bet, if you enjoy it. We recommend nonstrenuous dancing. Many dance instructors offer special exercises designed for laymen who wish to tone up. Dancing has the added advantage of being an enjoyable social activity.

Walking can't be beat. A leisurely walk, preferably in a quiet, pastoral setting, either alone or with a companion, will soothe your nerves and get oxygen to where it is needed. There is something about being outside in the night, especially if the air is clean and stars can be seen, that helps lift the cares of the day and restore a sense of perspective.

If you don't care to go out, or if it is too late, and you feel restive and a bit sluggish in .the limbs, just doing a few pushups, situps, or half-kneebends will help.

The Long Swing: One last exercise is highly recommended before bed for its relaxing effects, and for its marvelous influence on the eyes. An astounding amount of tension gets deposited in the muscles around the eyes. Eighty-six percent of our sensory input is visual, and much of the day we are straining or otherwise overstimulating the eyes. This exercise, developed by an ophthalmologist named W.H. Bates, and lauded by Aldous Huxley in *The Art of Seeing*, will relax your eye muscles and prevent you from "staring" in your dreams, a phenomenon that is said to cause headaches and eyestrain at night.

Stand with your feet comfortably apart and sway slowly from one foot to the other. Let your arms hang loosely, and keep your head straight, with your nose pointed straight ahead. Swing your body a full 180 degrees from right to left and back again, allowing hips, shoulders, head and eyes to swing easily together. Keep your eyes open and relaxed. Make no attempt to focus on anything. Breathe normally as you turn, in coordination with your swing. Swing easily, gracefully, and pleasurably, with your muscles loose.

While doing this, blink, somewhat more often than usual. You should swing at a rate of about 16 complete turns a minute, or once every four seconds. Practice this Long Swing for about five minutes before turning out the lights, and you should get to bed more relaxed.

Take a Bath Before Bed

A warm bath before retiring will help increase the circulation to the skin, which will make you sleepy. Prepare your bed before you bathe, perhaps while the tub is filling up. The water should be warm, never hot; body temperature is recommended. Never let the temperature of the water exceed 100 degrees F. or dip beneath 90. Fill it so you can immerse yourself in the water as fully as possible.

You may improve the soothing qualities of warm water by adding ordinary baking soda. This will make the bath more alkaline and benefit the nerves on the surface of the skin. A few drops of oil of eucalyptus can also be added. A tablespoon of mustard powder or genuine pine needle essence, will have a normalizing, relaxing effect on the body's circulation.

Immerse yourself for about 20 minutes. Close your eyes, dim the bathroom lights, and just let yourself unwind. Some soft music, such as the pieces suggested earlier, will add to the serene atmosphere.

After the bath, dry yourself by patting gently with a fluffy towel. Don't rub—the friction will be stimulating. Then go quietly to bed. *Do* go to bed though. We suggested this restful bath to a young lady named Jane Davis, and the next day when we asked her how it had worked, she said, "It worked too well. I fell asleep in the bath!"

John Lust, author of *The Herb Book*, recommends these full bath formulas for insomniacs:

1. Steep two ounces of balm leaves in a quart of boiling water for 15 minutes.

2. Add seven ounces of angelica root to two quarts of cold water, bring to a boil, and steep for five minutes.

3. Add three to four ounces of valerian root to one quart of cold water, let soak for ten to 12 hours, bring to a brief boil.

4. Steep three to four ounces of mother-of-thyme in one pint of boiling water for 10 minutes.

In each case add the concoction to your bath water.

Footbaths are also recommended, and two variations are offered:

1. Dip your feet and calves into a deep pot or a tub filled with cold water, keeping them in until the cold becomes uncomfortable or the feet feel warm.

2. Alternate between the hot herbal foot bath and the cold water, beginning with the hot for one to two minutes, followed by half a minute in the cold, and alternating in that manner for 15 minutes. End with the cold.

CHAPTER NINE

WHAT TO DO IN BED

In the dead of the night I am only one of the dark millions riding forward in black buses toward the unknown.

—F. Scott Fitzgerald

So it's time for bed. You've done everything you can to help yourself get to sleep. Now the question is, will you slip quietly into slumber, as nature intended, without having to resort to any more contrivances, or will you struggle yet another night?

If you have read the material in this book carefully, if you have given serious thought to your own sleep and your own life-style, and if you have applied the treatments recommended in a way that suits you, and if you have applied them diligently, you will probably be able to lie down when tired and drift off into a natural sound sleep. That, however, is the ideal. It will come, eventually. But in the meantime, and on those inevitable occasions when circumstances interfere, you will need techniques for encouraging sleep at the time you need it most.

There are many techniques that you can employ in bed. The one cardinal rule that you should follow in doing whatever you decide to do is, *"Trying is prohibited!"* The absolutely worst thing you can do for your sleep is to try.

Slumber represents a de-excited state, while the act of trying—even mildly—is an excited state. It activates the brain, and when it is time for sleep, arousal is the opposite of what you want. Bedtime is time to let go, not time to struggle. "Sleep, like the Kingdom of Heaven, is not taken by force," said one writer. Let sleep take you by force—be a willing captive.

This chapter offers plausible techniques for bringing about a receptive state of mind and body. Our personal recommendation is that you lean toward the physical methods over the mental ones. The mind is a delicate instrument, about which we know precious little. To manipulate it artificially seems to us as potentially dangerous as using untested drugs. It is too easy to fall into the mistake of trying too hard, especially when you are getting desperate for sleep. Trying will only add tension to the system and prevent sleep from coming naturally.

Physical techniques can relax mind and body with less likelihood of self-defeating strain. But even they must be put in proper perspective. Too many books on the subject, and too many insomniacs, make the mistake of relying exclusively on the types of techniques we will describe in this chapter. They are extremely important, and a vital part of your arsenal, but they are, in a sense, last resorts. As we said before, the best time to deal with your sleep problem is all day long, by learning how to live a healthy, happy, tension-free life. If the techniques in this chapter work for you, great. But, if your problem is severe or chronic, only the changes in patterns and habits brought about by the previously mentioned treatments will bring lasting results. In-bed practices should be done only when necessary.

Massage

For relieving muscular tension, and to just plain feel good, few procedures can rival a good massage. It will greatly improve circulation, particularly in the limbs, and prevent the stiffness and cramping that often interfere with sleep. If you are fortunate enough to have someone who will massage you before sleep, that is probably the best way to take advantage of massage, for you are then in the most passive state. *The Massage Book*, by George Downing, is the one to have for instructions on administering massage to another person.

Under the assumption that you do not have so cooperative a person around, and because you will want to use massage when it is dark and late and you have only yourself to rely on, we have selected a few relaxing massages that can be self-administered. You might want to precede your massage with a full bath, as prescribed in the previous chapter. After patting yourself dry, apply almond or coconut oil to your skin. Do this slowly and in a leisurely manner, without rubbing the skin coarsely.

Here is a good full-body massage you can do sitting up in bed:

• Begin with your hands on the top of your head. Press gently, but firmly with your palms and fingertips. Move forward slowly, pressing deeply, over the forehead and down over the face. Linger for a while at whatever points feel particularly good. Continue down over the throat and chest, stopping at the heart.

• Place your hands back on the top of your head. Again press and release (do not lift your hands, by the way; slide them along pressing as you go), this time going down the back of the head. Come down over the back of the neck, and across the shoulders. Give the neck and shoulder muscles lots of attention as they tend to gather considerable tension. Then come down over the top of the shoulders and across the chest.

• Now take your left hand and grasp the fingertips of the right hand. Press and release in the same manner, deeply and firmly but with a gentle motion, moving up the right arm, with your thumb on the underside and your fingers on top. Come all the way up to the shoulder, then down the chest to the heart. Now place your left thumb on the upper part of your right arm, and your fingers on the underside, and repeat the process. Switch arms, massaging your left arm both on top and underneath.

• Now place your hands on your belly, middle fingers touching at the navel. Massage your belly and abdomen very gently, then press and release as before, moving up the front of the body to the chest.

- Place your hands on your lower back, fingertips touching at the coccyx. Massage the back and sides, pressing and releasing until you reach as high as you can.
- Now for the all important feet and legs. Grasp the toes of your right foot with your hands, right hand on top and left underneath. Massage the toes and feet thoroughly. Now begin moving up the leg, over the ankle and calf, pressing and releasing deeply and thoroughly, but being careful not to cause discomfort or pain. Give your feet and calves as much time as you like, as circulation there is crucial. Come up over the knee and continue in like manner all the way up the thigh. If you care to recline to massage the legs, do so by all means. Lie on your back and bend your knee so you can reach the area you are massaging without having to reach too far. In some cases, you may not be able to massage from a reclining position until you get to your calf.

The upper parts of the body, particularly the face, are often the areas most in need of a bedtime massage. Here are some localized massages for those areas:

Head

- Place the index and middle fingers of both hands side by side on the top of your head and massage your scalp with deep pressure for about five seconds. Cover your whole scalp in this way. Now move your hands behind your head and place the index and middle fingers of both hands in the slight indentation at the center of the top of your neck, just below the base of the skull. Apply deep pressure for a few seconds, rotating the fingertips in a circular motion. Pause and repeat twice.
- Move your hands away from each other along the base of the skull about 1½ to two inches (or the width of two fingers), and apply deep pressure there with the index and middle fingers. Move your hands another inch or two and repeat the procedure at the point on the base of the skull adjacent to the ears.

Neck

- Place the index and middle fingers of your left hand at

the starting point (the top) of the large muscle that runs along the side of the neck from the base of the skull to the shoulder line. Place your right hand in the corresponding position on the other side. Apply deep pressure and massage these points thoroughly for a few seconds. Move your fingers slowly down the muscle lines to your shoulders, applying pressure along the way.

Shoulders

• There is a very tender spot slightly to the rear of your shoulder, at the point halfway between the base of the neck and the edge of the shoulder. Find that spot, and apply deep pressure with your fingertips and massage for a few seconds. Repeat a few times on both shoulders—this should go a long way toward removing tension in the shoulders, a key spot.

Upper back

• You will have to do some stretching to reach this one. Reach your left hand over your right shoulder as far down the right side of your spine as your arm can reach. Using your index, middle, and third fingers, apply deep pressure. Now move back up toward the shoulder, pausing at finger-widths to apply pressure. Repeat the sequence with your right hand on the left side of your spine.

Face

• This one can be done lying down. Close your eyes. Put both hands lightly over your face. Massage your forehead gently with your fingers in a slow, circular motion. Be very gentle with your face—neck and shoulders can be done more vigorously. Now slide your hands down a bit and repeat the circular movements, gently, over your eyelids and eye sockets.

• Slide your hands down still further, and, with your middle fingers at the corners of your mouth, stroke upward in light, circular movements. Go all the way up to the temples.

• Don't forget your scalp. Russian nobles had servants scratch their heads gently when insomnia threatened. The Japanese have a tradition of "skull massage" too. Use light, circular motions to massage the scalp with your fingertips.

Vibrators: There are many electronic aids to massage. We suggest using your hands, unless you find the vibrators particularly good for relieving extra-tense muscles. (We find the sound of the buzzing machine unsettling.) For the ultimate gadget you can purchase a device called a "Magic Fingers Bed Massager." It attaches to your bed, providing up to 30 minutes of massage at a time. It requires no special tools and is said to "convert any bed into a relaxing massager."

Foot Massage: Mrs. Kaufman suddenly found herself unable to sleep. The problem lasted for days and had everyone mystified—she had always been healthy and happy, and had always slept like a log the minute her head hit the pillow. While pondering the situation one day, she realized that the new shoes she had purchased were too tight. Intuitively, she felt there might be a connection. She returned the shoes for a looser, more comfortable pair. She felt better during the day. And she slept better at night. The constriction of her feet had caused the sort of fatigue that, ironically, prevents sleep from coming naturally.

There may be more to that story than mere coincidence or ordinary pain. Apparently, the various organs, nerves, and glands in our bodies are connected with certain "reflex areas" on the feet. Each specific organ has a known association with a particular point on the sole, toes, ankles or heel. For this reason, and because we often spend long hours standing and walking in shoes of questionable comfort, our feet are more important than we might imagine. For insomniacs, it is a wise idea to make sure the circulation in the feet is unobstructed.

Here is a foot massage excellent for relieving discomfort and improving circulation.

• Sit comfortably, with your left leg crossed over the right so that you can easily grasp the left foot. Using the knuckles of your right hand, massage the sole of the foot (you might use the eraser end of a pencil instead). Press firmly, moving in small circles. Cover the entire sole. Go slowly, and don't be squeamish. When you dig into a particularly tender area, you have probably located crystalline deposits on nerve endings. The tenderness is an indication that the area needs attention. Dig in, but be careful not to press hard on ligaments or tendons.

- After massaging the entire sole, go to the top of the foot. Using the tips of your thumbs (not the soft, fleshy pad, but the tips adjacent to the nail) cover the top of the foot from the toes to the ankle. As before, massage in a circular motion. On top of the foot, you should be gentle, but firm.
- Massage the bottom edge of the heel with your fingertips and thumb. Press hard.
- Along the top of your feet are long tendons that run from the base of the ankle down to each toe. Press firmly with the tip of your thumb in the valleys between tendons, and run the thumb down the foot to the toe. Do this in each valley.
- Grasp your foot with both hands, pressing your fingertips into the sole. The heels of your hands should touch on top of the foot. Press hard on top and bottom, and slide your hands out to the edges of the foot.
- Holding your foot steady with one hand, grasp the big toe with your thumb and forefinger. Pull gently, and shake the toe. Repeat with each toe.
- Repeat this entire process on your right foot.

For mechanical assistance in caring for the all-important feet, try the Songrand Footbath, a portable whirlpool bath that churns water around the feet. It is very refreshing, as is the Dr. Scholl's Foot Massager, a vibrating pad that you can rest your feet upon while seated for a complete massage.

Take care of your feet, and remember to avoid tight shoes. That often-heard lament in shoe stores—"But I've always worn a size six!"—has probably kept many a person awake.

Breathing Techniques

The significance of breathing is well expressed in this paragraph from the *Encyclopedia Britannica:*

> The conception of life is so closely bound up with that of respiration that the very word 'expiration' has come to connote the extinction of life, and 'inspiration' its elevation to a super-human level. Respiration is a process common to all forms of life, the reason for which is that the chemical basis of life is essentially an oxidation of tissue.

In our own culture and in the East, breathing techniques have been developed for achieving relaxation, improving digestion, and in other ways normalizing the body. Several of these are significant aids for insomniacs at bedtime.

The Kelly Method: When a person is asleep, there is an increase in the carbon dioxide level of the blood. This, coupled with the fact that carbon dioxide has a natural tranquilizing effect that often brings on drowsiness, led Dr. Charles Kelly to develop a program of controlled breathing that has been found to help people fall asleep. The techniques are designed to increase the carbon dioxide level of the blood. They are said to be easy, effective, and free from any possible side effects.

• Lie either on your back or on either side, whichever you find more conducive to easy breathing. Make sure your room is dark, and well-ventilated. Use a pillow that is just high enough to keep your head straight, or perhaps tilted slightly back. Be sure not to have the head lean forward— when it tilts slightly back the throat and eye muscles are relaxed, and breathing is freer.

• Close your eyes lightly.

• Begin with a few very deep inhalations, filling the lungs and expanding the chest as much as possible. Then exhale fully, drawing in the abdomen to expel as much air as possible. Repeat this three times.

• At the end of the third exhalation, when the lungs are as empty as possible, hold your breath for as long as you can. Hold it until the impulse to breathe cannot be resisted easily. Then repeat the three deep breaths, again holding your breath at the end of the third exhalation.

By doing this, you are gradually accumulating carbon dioxide in the body. The three deep breaths restore the oxygen content of the blood and remove enough carbon dioxide to allow the breath to be held longer, and therefore for more carbon dioxide to be produced. The carbon dioxide makes the chemical balance of the blood more acidic, and it slows the activity of the nerves and the brain, preparing them for the onset of natural sleep.

It is important, however, not to take more than three deep breaths in any part of the cycle, to keep the carbon dioxide buildup at just the right level. If you deviate from

Kelly's prescription, chances are the carbon dioxide will be eliminated and drowsiness will not come.

• When not breathing at the end of the third breath, keep the lungs as empty as possible to prevent the carbon dioxide from being absorbed from the bloodstream by the lungs.

Do not fear that you are being deprived of oxygen. You have more than enough in your bloodstream to nourish your cells, and as soon as you resume normal breathing, your body will balance itself accordingly.

• To aid the breath retention distract your mind from the effort by thinking of a song or a poem you can recite to yourself. Or you may prefer to use one of the other imagination-aids that we will discuss later.

• Turn your eyes upward during the breathing exercises, since it has been found that the position is conducive to sleep.

After perhaps five to eight periods of maximum deep breaths (three per set) and long breath-holding, you will feel a strong desire to breathe normally. You will also feel more relaxed and eager to rest. Quite possibly you will have fallen asleep before you do this five times.

If, after eight repetitions, you still cannot fall asleep, try the following exercise. Do not use it, however, until you have mastered the first.

In this exercise you will again take in as deep a breath as you can, and exhale as much air as you can. Again, do this three times. After the third, however, instead of holding your breath, you will have a period of what Kelly calls "minimum breathing."

"Minimum breathing," says Kelly, "means breathing in and out so slightly that the movement of the air in the nostrils is just perceptible. The minimum breathing must be very shallow and the breaths very short."

• Do not fill the lungs with air. Keep the abdomen completely relaxed—don't tense the muscles. Do this until you feel the urge to breathe more deeply. Then start another series of three maximally deep breaths and complete expulsions. After those three, repeat the minimum breathing again.

• Continue in this manner as long as necessary, and as long as it is comfortable. Remember not to strain. Be casual. You will find your mind drifting so much you will forget how many breaths you have taken, or maybe even what you are doing in the first place. That is fine. Don't regret such events, and don't strain to remain alert for the purpose of doing the exercise. The purpose, remember, is to do the opposite—drift into oblivion. Indeed, this technique can often be so effective you will drift off during the minimum breathing periods.

Remember to take "rest" periods of normal breathing between repetitions. And don't be discouraged if neither exercise works the first few times. We have found the Kelly method to be quite effective whenever we are agitated. It is also very helpful upon awakening during the night.

Alternate Nostril Breathing: This is a traditional Yoga practice, customarily done before periods of meditation. It is remarkably calming, and is said to restore equilibrium to the nervous system. Do it sitting up in bed comfortably (if awakened in the night, you might find it helpful to just do it lying there).

• Place the tip of your right thumb against your right nostril. Place the middle and ring fingers against your left nostril. Keep your hand relaxed. Close the right nostril with the thumb and breath in through the left.

• Inhale slowly and easily with the body relaxed. The breath may be slightly deeper than usual, but make no effort to take in an extra quantity of air. Some sources recommend holding the breath for three or four seconds once it is inhaled. We have found that, when drowsy, such an attempt might be a strain. Let's keep it optional.

• When ready, exhale. But exhale through the *right* nostril, lifting the thumb and closing the left nostril with your other fingers. Exhale slowly, noiselessly, but without straining to go at any particular pace. Follow whatever pace is comfortable. (Some recommend inhaling and exhaling to a particular count—again, when drowsiness is being encouraged, this might cause strain.)

• After having exhaled, and perhaps held the breath momentarily, inhale through the right nostril, keeping the left one closed. When you have inhaled and feel the urge to exhale, switch nostrils, closing the right once again.

• The sequence, then, is as follows: out—in—switch nostrils—out—in—switch nostrils—out—in—switch nostrils. . .

You should do this alternate nostril technique for about five minutes. After you are accustomed to it, and it feels natural, you may increase to ten minutes, when necessary. Do not exceed ten minutes. Naturally, if you feel sufficiently drowsy, stop, lie down, and sleep.

If, at any point, you forget which nostril it is time to close, or whether to inhale or exhale, or if you forget for the moment why your fingers are at your nose, then the technique is working. You are likely to be drifting off into sleep.

There are no formal studies of these controlled breathing techniques, but the anecdotal evidence is substantial. That alternate-nostril breathing is a valuable aid in achieving relaxation is evidenced by its centuries of use in the Yoga tradition, and its increasing use in the West.

In our questioning of people who have tried many different techniques to improve their sleep, both the breathing practices described here have been given support. They can only help. If you do them some night and you still do not fall asleep easily, don't discard the techniques. It may have been a particularly bad night.

Hypnosis

Discovered in the eighteenth century by the Viennese doctor Franz Mesmer, modern hypnosis has had a stormy history. It was not until 1958 that the American Medical Association accepted hypnosis, provided it was done by trained doctors. Now it is widely used, by hypnotists who may or may not be M.D.'s, to help overcome specific phobias, fears, and unwanted habits. Not everyone can be hypnotized—it requires a certain amount of faith in the hypnotist, and the determination to do what he suggests. Even at that, some subjects are more susceptible than others. If you would like to try putting yourself in the hands of a hypnotist, keep in mind the following pros and cons:

• Direct suggestion is said to help calm the fear of not being able to fall asleep, which often is a self-fulfilling fear. It is also said to counteract apprehension and to foster the will to sleep. And it can restore confidence to the insomniac who has come to wonder if he will ever be able to sleep again.

• On the other hand, hypnosis does involve a certain

amount of surrender of will power. There is a chance you will become dependent on the hypnotist, or on the subterfuge of suggestion—which, it has been argued, is unnatural—and be unable to fall asleep any other way.

One person we interviewed, a bookkeeper-housewife named Shirley Todd, swears by her hypnosis. "I tried all sorts of things to help me sleep," she said. "Finally I went to a doctor who recommended a hypnotist. I was afraid at first; I didn't want to put myself in the hands of a stranger. But he quickly won my confidence. I had previously made up my mind that I'd never sleep without pills again. He practically bet me that he could put me to sleep. And he did. Right in his office. He shut the lights, and told me to relax. I can't recall his exact words, but he told me, basically, that I was getting tired—he used words like heavy, floating, drifting, and so on. At first I giggled, but after a while I was dozing off. Next thing I knew, he was waking me up from a deep nap. He gave me a tape to play before bed, with essentially the same sort of suggestions on it. It works."

Not all hypnotists use tapes, of course, although they are becoming quite the rage. Most often, the hypnotist will induce the trancelike state deemed necessary for implanting the suggestion, in his office. The suggestion having been made, it should trigger the conditioned reaction at the appropriate time.

The form of hypnosis many nonsleepers try to employ is the do-it-yourself style, known as self-hypnosis, or autosuggestion. One of the most famous examples of this appears in the writings of the French scientist, Emile Coué, who invented the familiar self-suggestion refrain, "Day by day, in every way, I grow better and better."

Coué wrote: "Every night when you have comfortably settled yourself in bed, you will repeat (not gobble), 'I am going to sleep, I am going to sleep,' in a quiet, placid, even voice, avoiding of course the slightest mental effort to obtain the result. The soporific effect of this droning repetition soon makes itself felt, whereas, if one actually tries to sleep, the spirit of wakefulness is kept alive by the negative idea, according to the law of converted effort."

Coué's method is basically the one used—in a thousand variations—by modern advocates of self-suggestion. They have certain things in common. The suggestions, it is said, should always be framed in a permissive, positive tone, such as "I can," "I will," or "I am going to." They all state that instant results should not be expected, as it often takes some time for the suggestions to be implanted in the subconscious mind. Also, suggestion is not the same as a command—don't issue orders to yourself, as though you could be forced to obey. Since confidence is an absolute must, self-hypnotists are advised not to attempt big objectives at the beginning. Start simple and work your way up. Never use the word "try" in your suggestions. And never use negatively phrased suggestions, such as "I am not going to stay awake."

In a sense, self-suggestion is something we all do much of the time. We are always telling ourselves, or trying to convince ourselves, that we are going to do something, or change something, or turn over a new leaf of some kind. The problem with self-hypnosis and sleep is that the will power that we usually try to induce through suggestion may increase our determination, but it may also keep us awake by inducing that enemy of sleep, trying.

Here is one example of a suggested form of self-hypnosis that we received from a self-employed hypnotist who wished to remain anonymous:

"Lie on your back in bed, with your arms at your side and your hands open. The room should be dark and quiet. Breathe deeply for two minutes, mentally saying to yourself, 'I will soon be fast asleep.' Then concentrate on the following suggestions. Repeat them for about five minutes: 'I am very comfortable, so very comfortable. My arms are heavy. My feet are heavy. My eyes are heavy. Everything is slowing down. I am floating and drifting. I want to fall asleep. I am beginning to fall asleep.' Repeat these, or words like them, and soon the feelings they describe will be felt, and you should fall asleep."

The hypnotist said that there are countless variations on that theme, including repeating the suggestions to the rhythm of deep breathing, and doing them along with techniques for muscle relaxation such as the Jacobson methods.

That should give you an idea of what is involved in self-hypnosis. We cannot vouch for any particular technique, although it is certainly plausible that they can, in fact, help induce sleep. Certainly, our minds are capable of exerting their will over our bodies and hypnosis certainly works for many other ailments. What we wonder about, is whether the state induced by hypnosis is natural sleep, and whether the suggestions ever become anything more than sophisticated self-deception.

Keep in mind the following opinions of medical authorities.

"In hypnosis," says Dr. Peter Steincrohn, an expert on relaxation, "the typical brain-wave changes observed during normal sleep do not occur, the knee-jerk reflex still operates, and the usual falls in blood pressure and pulse rate do not take place."

Most doctors seem to agree that the trance obtained in hypnosis or self-hypnosis is not the same as natural sleep. Says French doctor, Paul Chauchard, Director of the *Ecole des Hautes Etudes* in Paris, "Hypnotists work by paralyzing the part of the nerve center (in the brain) that controls sleep, but their method does not promote normal sleep. The sensitive nerve mechanisms are merely thrown out of action by upsetting their inner metabolism. This does not bring true repose."

If you choose to try hypnosis, remember it does not work for everyone. You should consult with an experienced clinical hypnotist to see if you are a likely candidate. Your local medical society, the psychiatry department of your local hospital, or the psychology department of your local university should be able to recommend reliable therapists who use hypnosis.

Relaxation Techniques

The literature on sleep contains a great number of relaxation exercises designed to reduce tension at bedtime. Many of these border on self-suggestion, much like the ones described in our section on hypnosis. Others are variations on the corpse pose, described in our section on Yoga, where the person wills each part of his body to relax progressively. Still others are variations on Jacobson's Progressive Relaxation techniques.

We screened these, and offer the ones that require a minimum of mental effort. They are easy to do and have a relatively immediate impact on muscular tension.

We recommend that, once you turn off the lights and lie down, you just lie there. Just be easy, don't do anything in particular, mentally or physically, and see what happens. If, after five or ten minutes, you feel tension in the muscles that does not seem to be diminishing, or is getting worse, then and only then should you use these techniques. It is better to give nature a chance on its own, without your involvement.

When you use these techniques (or any others for that matter), be extremely casual. Be nonchalant. Do not attempt to concentrate. If your mind drifts, let it go. It might be going to sleep. If you forget the sequence of exercises, or if you forget where you were because your mind wandered, don't get upset. Just do these innocently, and stop whenever you start drifting toward sleep.

The Steincrohn method:

• Lying on your back in a dark, quiet room, first clench your right fist tightly, and raise it off the bed with all muscles tensed. Hold for about a minute. Then let the arm go limp and drop it to the bed. After a minute, repeat this with the other arm. This time, let the tension *gradually* decrease until the arm is completely limp.

• Next, push both toes downward as far as they will go. Hold for a minute. Then suddenly stop the tension. Repeat the tensing, but this time let it decrease very gradually.

• Third, relax your chest by breathing in more deeply than usual. Hold your breath. Then let your chest go suddenly limp. Again, repeat this a few times, relaxing the muscles gradually.

• Now the forehead and face. Raise your forehead and relax it. Then lower the forehead in a frown and relax it. Repeat with gradual relaxing.

• Next the eyes. Look as far as you can toward your right ear (remember your eyes are closed) and hold for half a minute. Relax, wait a moment, and look toward your left ear. Again hold, then relax. Next, look up toward your hairline, hold half a minute, then relax. Finally, look toward your chin, hold half a minute, and relax.

• The last area is the speech area. Count out loud to ten. Notice the tension produced in the throat, lips, tongue and face. Relax all those muscles. Repeat the count, using less and less muscle movement, and saying it softer and softer.

Then do it again, trying not to use the speech muscles at all.

After a while, says Dr. Steincrohn, the full range of muscles should be triggered into relaxation in a moment.

Dr. Pai's method:

Dr. N. M. Pai, a staunch opponent of the use of sleeping pills long before it became fashionable to speak out on the matter, advocates what he calls the "tenlax" method:

• Lie comfortably on your back in a quiet, dark room, eyes closed. Tense your muscles by stretching your legs, and pointing your toes away from you. Pressing the back downward, hold your legs as long as you can in as tense a position as possible. Let go suddenly. After a moment, repeat the procedure. Do this six times.

• Then tense the muscles of your arms, clenching the fists as tightly as you can. Hold for as long as it is not unbearable. Let go suddenly. Repeat this six times.

• Eyes still closed, focus as though you were looking at the end of your nose. Then focus on your hairline.

Dr. Pai believes this series of maneuvers should be enough to lower anxiety in most people.

For those who have been chronically sleep-deprived, and who have been taking pills for it, Dr. Pai recommends the following:

• In the same setting and position, close off one nostril and exhale through the other. Then inhale. Switch nostrils, exhale and inhale, and switch again, alternately.

• While doing this, tense your leg muscles, pointing your toes, and lifting the legs slightly. Hold the legs in that manner for as long as you can. Then let go, dropping the legs.

• Discontinue the alternate breathing, and breathe normally. Clench your fists, hold for 20 seconds, and let go. Wait half a minute. Then raise your head and shoulders off your bed and hold for 20 seconds. Let go.

• Back to the legs. Stretch your right leg, pointing the toes. Tense the whole leg and hold it off the bed for 15 seconds. Let go. Switch legs and repeat. Continue to do this, alternating legs, a total of four times.

• Back to the arms. Clench your fists. Bend your elbows completely, with the arm muscles tense, and hold for as long as you can while simultaneously holding your breath. Let go.

Take a deep breath and relax completely, turning your eyes upward.

After a few lessons, says Dr. Pai, many of his patients slept soundly from then on. While doing any of Dr. Pai's exercises, stop as soon as you feel you are near falling asleep.

One more technique: There are countless varieties, as we said. Here is one derived from the Yoga tradition:

- Lie in bed on your back. Raise your right arm above your head so that it is in a straight line with your body. Stretch your right side from toes to fingers. Notice the feeling of tension, while reaching as far as you can. Then release. After a moment, repeat the process on your left side.
- Now stretch the nape of your neck and pull in your chin. Let go.
- Now put your palms on top of your head and pull backwards for half a minute.
- Stretch your face muscles, then let go.
- Open your mouth as wide as you can, then release. Repeat that a few times.
- Now hold your tongue against the side of your cheek for ten seconds. (See below.) Release. Bug your eyes out for ten seconds. Relax.
- Now massage each finger and thumb, shake your hands up and down and sideways. Bend the arm over the chest, clenching your fist. Tense the whole arm, then relax. Repeat, alternating arms, a few times.
- Pulling your toes toward you, press your legs against each other hard. Hold for a minute or more, then relax. Repeat this until you notice the absence of tension in your legs.
- Now expand your chest as much as possible, hold for a few seconds, and let go, exhaling slowly. Repeat until you feel relaxed in the chest muscles. Then exhale, pulling in your stomach as far as possible. Hold a few seconds and let go. Repeat several times.

Now yawn and go to sleep.

The tongue-in-cheek method: Dr. Steincrohn observed that his insomniac patients often pressed hard against the roofs of their mouths or against the back ridge of their upper teeth. He suggests ways to relax the important muscles around the jaw. Let your tongue relax by pulling it away from the roof of your mouth or the back of your teeth, and gently slide it between your teeth, against the inner cheek. Hold this for a few minutes. It should help you relax.

Dr. Steincrohn claims that this simple method is the most effective device he knows for relieving tension-related insomnia.

Roll Up Your Eyes

On the battlefields of World War I, a fortuitous discovery was made by the famous neurologist, Dr. Foster Kennedy. The Fifth British Army was retreating. Dr. Kennedy saw soldiers so exhausted that they fell on the ground where they were and plunged into a sleep as deep as a coma. They didn't even wake up when the doctor raised their eyelids with his fingers.

It was when he was raising those eyelids that Dr. Kennedy made his serendipitous discovery. Invariably, the pupils of the soldiers' eyes were rolled upwards in their sockets. "After that," Dr. Kennedy wrote, "when I had trouble sleeping, I would practice rolling up my eyeballs into this position, and I found that in a few seconds I would begin to yawn and feel sleepy. It was an automatic reflex over which I had no control."

Since then Dr. Kennedy's observation has been confirmed. Experiments have shown that we always fall asleep with our eyes in an upward position.

Whatever the explanation—some have suggested fatigue of the eye muscles, for example—keeping the eyes upward by looking over the head (eyes closed of course) will often help bring on sleep.

You might even start the process with the eyes open. Stare at a spot behind your head so that your eyes are required to rise to the top of the sockets. Open and close the eyes in this position a few times, then keep them closed for sleep.

Here is another technique for the eyes, advocated by Aldous Huxley in his *Art of Seeing*. Warm your hands by rubbing them briskly together. Now place the palms lightly over your eyes with the sides of your hands against the sides of your nose. Don't exert pressure on your eyeballs, but keep all light from entering your eyes. A minute or two of this warming, soothing influence on the eyes can be remarkably calming.

What To Do About Leg Jitters

In chapter four we described an illness known as nocturnal myoclonus. It is often associated with similar jerking of the legs during wakefulness. Known as leg jitters, this condition prevents the person from keeping the legs still while lying down to sleep. It is quite common, occurring on and off for many insomniacs.

The earliest known description of this condition was made by the great clinical neurologist, Dr. Thomas Willis, in 1695: "Wherefore to some, when being a Bed they betake themselves to sleep, presently in the Arms and Leggs, Leapings and Contractions of the Tendons, and so great a Restlessness and Tossings of their Members ensue, that the diseased are no more able to sleep, than if they were in a Place of the greatest Torture."

Modern sufferers of leg jitters have described the sensations involved in various ways—as creeping, pulling, or stretching inside the leg itself. Some have said it felt as though the leg were filled with worms or ants. In some cases the jerking, which has been described as "diabolical," may last several hours, during which time it is impossible to fall asleep.

The exact cause of restless legs is uncertain. There are indications that it is associated with a vitamin deficiency or anemia. Taking iron pills is said to help, especially during the last third of pregnancy, when as many as ten percent of women report having some experience of restless legs. Regular large doses of ascorbic acid (vitamin C) is also said to be helpful.

Doctors have given patients vasodilator drugs for a month or more, in order to relieve the condition. The creeping sensation has been relieved by drugs such as Priscoline, Ronical, and Carbrital.

Dr. Steincrohn, whom we have quoted several times, claims that an effective treatment for leg jitters is to soak in a hot bath, and do ten deep knee-bends afterwards. Aspirin may help also.

If you have this condition recurrently, and if none of the above suggestions work, see your doctor or go to the nearest sleep clinic.

Point Your Head in the Right Direction

Baron Charles de Reichenbach, the inventor of paraffin, used to say that in cases of insomnia, the person should simply turn around and sleep with his head at the foot of the bed.

We don't know if the Baron's method worked or not, but, if the insomniac happened to be pointing in the wrong direction, it just may have. From all the cardinal points have come folk stories about the magnetic effects of pointing your head in a certain direction. Charles Dickens, for example, would not go anywhere without a compass. He insisted on sleeping with his head pointed north, and would move the furniture around over the protests of innkeepers.

As soon as Ben Franklin's kite demonstrated the reality of electromagnetism, millions of Americans rushed out to buy magnets to help realign the electromagnetic energies in their bodies.

Studies of men in the polar regions of the earth have shown that sleep is more difficult there. Despite their heavy work, few of the men studied had any Stage IV sleep. When they returned to their homelands, it took a full year to reestablish their previous sleep patterns. According to a government study, the reason for this aberration was the magnetic field at the pole.

Other studies have demonstrated the effects of magnetic fields on the emotions. A Canadian study, for example, showed that mental patients had periods of extreme mobility and increased disorientation whenever there were large magnetic changes from the weather, or sunspots.

Dr. E. B. Foote insisted in 1870 that, at night, the magnetic and electric currents of the earth predominate, markedly influencing sleep.

The question is, which direction is the right direction? Dickens insisted it was north, as do many others. However, according to certain Yogic traditions, north is the *least* desirable direction in which to face, and east is the choice.

Try to sleep with your head toward the north for a few nights; then try it toward the east. Vary directions every few nights to see if any one has an effect on your sleep. You may find, as many have, that direction makes the difference.

The Best Position To Sleep In

There is an old Islamic proverb that says: only kings may sleep on the right side; the left side is for wise men; saints may sleep on their backs; and it's the devil's privilege to sleep on his stomach.

In our own culture, psychologists have recently taken to studies of our favorite sleeping postures. Dr. Samuel Dunkell, author of the amusing, *The Sleep Position: The Night Language of the Body*, claims that "a preferred sleeping position is stubbornly clung to because it expresses how we feel about the world." Dunkell describes an amazing range of positions with clever names like flamingo, monkey, cyclops, sphinx, chain gang, and swastika. He says, for example, that sleeping flat on the back in what he calls the *royal* posture, expresses openness and unusual confidence.

Whatever the underlying unconscious reasons, your position in bed does make a difference in how well you sleep. For one thing, faulty posture may cause physical problems, to which you might ascribe the wrong cause. J. I. Rodale, founder of *Prevention* magazine, told of his experience in eliminating a persistent neuritis when he realized that he laid his head on his arm during sleep. The pressure was pinching nerves. There is also the danger of cutting off circulation to parts of the body, which will either awaken you or make your sleep inefficient.

Most experts counsel against sleeping on your stomach—it is not good for the neck muscles, or for breathing. Lying on the back is not the top choice, but is superior to lying on your stomach. If you lie on your back, you might try placing a pillow or two under your knees. Or, purchase one of several wedge-shaped pillows made specifically for that purpose, at a sleep shop. Some people advocate the use of bed blocks, or decks—wooden or plastic wedges that raise the mattress at the foot of the bed (or at the head of the bed, for reading). Said to aid circulation, these devices have the added advantage of discouraging you from lying on your stomach.

The ideal position for sleeping is pictured in drawing. In it, the spine is in a straight line; the knees and elbows are relaxed, with the limbs free of the body; the body is anchored by the bones, not by the pull of muscles; shoulders and hips are anchored. This position gives you lots of freedom for the 20 to 35 position changes we each make during the night.

The hands and feet can be moved to positions that are comfortable for your particular build. A thin pillow may be placed under the uppermost knee, if you like.

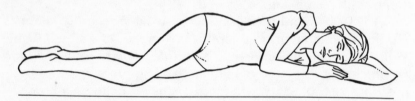

Remember, that while this may be the ideal position, and has the endorsement of sleep experts and posture specialists like Dr. James McDonnell, you have been accustomed to a different position for a long time. It may take a while to readjust. Also, you will find yourself falling back on your old postures during the night. Take your time retraining yourself.

"I had always slept on my stomach," said insomniac Charlie Clarke, "and I had neck problems all my life. When I finally connected the two, I tried to sleep on my side. It was virtually impossible, at first anyway. Then I decided to go about it systematically. I started out by lying on my side, and I stayed in that position until I couldn't stand it any longer. I kept a foggy eye on the clock, and tried to extend the time a little bit each night—maybe a minute or two. It took weeks before I could fall asleep in that position, but finally I did. I also found myself lying on my stomach in the middle of the night. When I caught myself, I turned over on my side—*if* it was no great strain. Gradually, I kicked the habit of sleeping on my stomach, and both my neck and my sleep improved."

Mark Twain had some characteristic advice about sleep position: "If you can't sleep, try lying on the end of the bed—then you might drop off."

Use Your Imagination

How do people go to sleep? I'm afraid I've lost
the knack. I might try busting myself smartly
over the temple with the nightlight. I might
repeat to myself, slowly and soothingly, a list of
quotations beautiful from minds profound; if I
can remember any of the damn things.
—character from a Dorothy Parker story

A good many people advocate the use of mind games,
such as repeating "a list of quotations beautiful from minds
profound," to court sleep. Others feel that such exercises only
keep the mind active, and are therefore antagonistic to sleep.
We tend to agree with the latter view. You can get so caught
up in a mind game that you will struggle to keep awake just to
complete it, or to get to the bottom of some perplexing puzzle
you have contrived.

With that thought in mind, we should also mention that
mind games have been found useful, if not for inducing
sleep, then at least for keeping the mind on relatively
cheerful distractions when it might otherwise get bogged
down in worries, especially worries over losing sleep. "The
chief virtue of brain games," writes Hilary Rubinstein, author
of the delightful, *Insomniacs of the World, Goodnight*, "is
that they keep the mind occupied in a psychologically harmless way. . . . I find that a session of compiling crossword
clues, for instance, makes me much less of a tosser and turner
than worrying about work, and sooner or later, my mind has
had enough of its early morning exercise, and I drop off once
again."

There is, of course, an infinite variety of things to
imagine, scenes to create, games to play, puzzles to solve, and
fantasies to indulge in. Some people like to imagine being on
some tropical island swimming, or fishing, or to imagine any
other idyllic scene that gives them a good memory or a good
expectation.

Visualizing a favorite person, recalling times of great joy
or love, or projecting some anticipated scene of the same
nature, are also favorites. Many of them get quite personal.
One very sound sleeper we know, sportswriter Clark Hanson,
told us his secret:

"As soon as I close my eyes, I imagine a baseball scene. It is usually the last inning of the last game of the World Series. It's two out, the score is tied, and the bases are loaded. I am either the centerfielder or the relief pitcher just brought in from the bullpen. If I'm in center field, the batter hits a tremendous fly ball that I overhaul by leaping to the top of a ten-foot fence, catching it just before the ball reaches the stands. If I'm the relief pitcher, I strike the batter out. Then, after leaving the field to the appreciative roar of the crowd, I lead off the bottom of the ninth with a game-winning home run. I usually fall asleep before I get to the locker room for the champagne party."

Mr. Hanson says he has been falling asleep to that tune ever since he was ten years old.

Some people need a more protective fantasy to overcome the fears of the night. Here is one from an anonymous science writer: around the edge of her bed she arranges a squadron of protective jungle beasts, all on guard, facing outward, keeping a watchful eye on the door to her room.

Others do things that border on self-hypnosis, like imagining that their hands, arms, legs, and feet are slowly turning to lead.

Lewis Carroll used to invent mathematical games to counter his insomnia. In 1888, he published a book called *Curiosa Mathematica*, which had a section entitled "Pillow Problems."

Spelling words backwards; naming towns, countries, baseball players, authors, or anything else going in order from A to Z; plotting a trip across the country to see if you know the map; naming the capital city of every state; casting a movie with famous actors playing your friends and family; naming every city (country, author, movie star, etc.) that begins with the letter q, z, or y.

The possibilities are endless, of course. Invent your own to suit your needs. If worse comes to worse, there is always counting sheep.

You might try a new technique of imagination that has had some clinical success. Anees A. Sheikh, a psychology professor at Marquette University, developed the technique, based on the principles of Eidetic Psychotherapy. First, the individual is asked to recall past occasions when he was fatigued but had to fend off sleep because of external demands—studying for an exam, working late, a long motor trip, etc.

Professor Sheikh has his patients recall the situation and concentrate on the mental image. The person becomes drowsy. He is then told to disregard the demand that forced him to stay awake in the original instance. In this way he reverses the results and falls asleep instead of remaining awake as he did in the earlier situation.

Dr. Sheikh advises experimentation with different images, and settling on one that works. It must be a real situation, not a hypothetical one.

What To Do About Snoring

Reportedly, one of every eight Americans snores. That means that on any given night over 25 million snorers are competing with the hoot owls and nightingales, sending out a dissonant drone that is probably keeping a good percentage of the remaining would-be sleepers awake. While snoring is the subject of a great many jokes, it is no laughing matter to the person who sleeps in the same room with a snorer. Snoring has been the cause of torment in honeymoon suites, college dormitories, and army barracks throughout the world. And the sad thing about it is: it hurts only those who hear it, not those who do it.

What is snoring? Most descriptions of it say that it is caused by air going past the soft palate and the uvula, the soft piece of tissue that hangs down the back of the throat. Some experts attribute snoring to nasal obstructions caused by enlarged adenoids or tonsils, deviate nasal septums, polyps, allergies, or excessive smoking and drinking. Another explanation is that, when lying on the back (the position in which most snoring occurs) the back of the person's tongue might fall against the throat walls, forming a kind of mechanical constriction that causes the tongue and throat tissues to vibrate.

What can you do about an inveterate snorer? If it's possible, sleep in a separate room. If not, wear ear plugs, or, train yourself to ignore the snoring. Better yet, get the person to stop. There is a wide range of techniques—practical and ludicrous—that may be tried.

- Wake the person each time he or she begins to snore. Perhaps rig up a buzzer under the pillow that you can operate without stirring. This takes persistence and dedication.
- Have the snorer adjust his or her sleeping position, so as to discourage breathing through the mouth. Some examples: sleep on the side with the forearm under the chin to keep the mouth closed; or place the upper arm over the extended lower arm, and cup the hand under the chin. If the snorer must sleep on his or her back, place a small pillow under the nape of the neck; or, place a small pillow under the chin, held in place by an elastic strap or an arm, to keep the mouth closed.
- To prevent turning over onto the back, place pillows in the way.
- During the Revolutionary War, soldiers sewed a pocket on the back of their nightclothes and inserted a ball or block of wood to discourage turning over onto the back. Have the snorer do something like that. Sleep shops sell a small ball to be attached to pajamas, à la revolutionary soldier.
- Try increasing the humidity in the room. Membranes swollen from too much dryness can cause snoring.
- Snorers might reduce intake of cheese, milk and bread. These can cause a build-up of mucus that could obstruct breathing.
- Get the snorer to lose weight. Obese persons are more prone to snoring.
- An important thing for an habitual snorer to do is to see an ear, nose and throat specialist. If some obstruction in the nose is the cause of the snoring, it can be cured by medical treatment—nose drops, sprays or antihistamines, for example—or surgery designed to open up the passages for free breathing.

Why Not Get Up And Do Something?

Leave your bed upon the first desertion of sleep; it being ill for the eyes to read lying, and worse for the mind to be idle; since the head during laziness is commonly a cage for unclean thoughts.

—Francis Osborn, English writer

The bed is for sleeping in. The more you limit its function to just that, many psychologists insist, the better you will sleep. Behavioral psychologists like Richard R. Bootzin of Northwestern University, have devised a simple method of overcoming what Bootzin calls the "misuse of bed."

The problem, according to Dr. Peter Hauri, is that many persons who have had periods of insomnia come to hate the night because they dread not being able to sleep. Then, of course, these people cannot sleep because that dread makes them too tense. "In this kind of case," says Dr. Hauri, "the individual has, somewhere along the line, become conditioned to his bedtime environment. The pillow, the bed, the lamp, etc., are not cues for drowsiness but for increased alertness and arousal. And so he starts tossing and turning."

One answer to the problem is Bootzin's regimen for reconditioning the person to those bedtime conditions that have been signals for tension and wakefulness. The patient is told to go to bed only when tired, and to get out of bed if sleep does not come in ten minutes. Staying there any longer is to misuse the bed, which, he must relearn, is only for sleeping. In no uncertain terms, the patient is told that he may not lie in it after that ten minutes; he must leave the room entirely, and think about his problems away from the bedroom environment.

The patients are told they can only return to the bedroom when they think they can fall asleep. They must continue this cycle of going to bed and getting up until they fall asleep, never remaining in bed longer than ten minutes. In addition, patients are to set an alarm for the same time every morning, including weekends, and must not oversleep, even if sleep does not come until a few minutes before the alarm goes off.

According to Hauri, "On the first night of this treatment, the patient usually won't sleep at all; he'll feel miserable the whole day after. But the following night, being tired, he'll get off to sleep somewhere about 3:00 or 4:00 in the morning. The night after that he stays awake for something like three hours. The next night it might be two. And then the individual gets happy, because he sees that it's going to work. Within about two to three weeks, many chronic insomniacs can be retrained in this way so that they can just hit the pillow and fall asleep."

This reconditioning procedure, needless to say, requires

a good deal of fortitude. Getting out of bed, even if you can't sleep, can be a miserable experience at 4:00 in the morning. "Most often a patient will need someone behind him, some sleep or behavioral therapist, to hold his hand and tell him that he's doing fine and that things are sure to get better," Hauri says.

Even if your case is not severe enough to warrant such a rigorous procedure, you might be wise to get out of bed when it becomes clear that sleep is not on its way. If nothing else, you might be wasting time. And time is the one thing that you can't make up—even sleep loss can be redeemed.

"The most important thing in bed," says Dr. Joseph Mendels, a sleep researcher, "is not to toss and turn. If you are restless, sit up, turn the lights on, and read for a while, or get up and do something else. Tossing and turning tends to aggravate the cycle of not sleeping—you become more tense and make the situation worse."

Use the time. You will be surprised how much you can accomplish in those quiet hours. Alexander Dumas, author of *The Three Musketeers*, was a notorious insomniac who tried all manner of cures until a famous doctor told him to get out of bed when he couldn't sleep. Dumas would wander the streets of town, watch the sunrise from a hill, or stroll along a river—predawn excursions that inspired some lovely prose. His anxiety relieved, Dumas eventually slept soundly through the night.

Robert Louis Stevenson was another author who began to enjoy nighttime expeditions. "I have not often enjoyed a more serene possession of myself, nor felt more independent of material aids," said Stevenson of his nights spent outdoors. "We have a moment to look upon the stars. And there is a special pleasure for some minds in the reflection that we share the impulse with all outdoor creatures in our neighborhood, that we have escaped out of the Bastille of civilisation, and are become, for the time being, a mere kindly animal and a sheep of Nature's flock."

Remember when you were a child, and your parents made you go to sleep? Remember how you protested? And remember how little it bothered you then to be unable to fall asleep, or to awaken early? You talked to your toys, you imagined marvelous adventures, you sorted out your baseball cards or tidied up your dollhouse. You enjoyed a rare moment of privacy. Sleep was a nuisance. What happened? Try to recapture the happiness of the waking state and you will probably make better use of the fact that you can't sleep. You may even come to count it as a blessing in disguise.

Now that we have electricity at our disposal, twentieth century insomniacs can do pretty much anything at night that they can do during the day. You need not have a great imagination to occupy yourself if you are reasonably alert. You may even come up with creative ideas that might not come during the hustle-bustle of the day. Indeed, the authors of this book think that its most inspired passages are those that dawned before dawn.

How about a trip outdoors? The air is fresher, the streets are quieter, at night than they are during the day. Of course, if you live in a city, the "outdoor creatures in our neighborhood," to which Stevenson referred, may be somewhat more unsavory, and so you may not want to go out alone. How about forming an insomniac's club? By way of precedent, a New York city ecology club called Friends of the Parks, has sponsored "insomniac bicycle tours" for the last eight years. Think of it—no autos, no crowds. "It's the only way we can pause and enjoy the great public environment—the cityscape," said founder Robert M. Makla. "You just can't do it in the middle of the day."

In 1977, the group expanded its range. It boarded a chartered train and descended on Washington, D.C. at 2:30 A.M., unloaded its bicycles, and toured the nation's capital until 8:00.

So, if you can't lick insomnia, join it. "It is at night," wrote Brian Aldiss, "that the mind is most clear, that we are most able to hold all our life in the palm of our skull."

Miscellaneous Tidbits

• Some have recommended placing a hot water bottle on your stomach and resting the insides of your wrists against it.
• Some habitual worriers claim to have solved the problem of worrying about tomorrow late into tonight by keeping a pad and pencil at bedside and writing down everything they are going to do the next day. They claim it stops them

from ruminating continuously. Writing things down has a sort of formality that fosters the making of definite decisions.

• If sinus pains keep you awake, or if clogged nostrils prevent you from breathing through your nose, thus waking you up, try using the unique Winco Electric Sinus Mask. It fits comfortably over the face with a window for complete vision. Says the catalogue, "gentle, measured penetrating heat eases congestion, pressures and pain."

• Van Gogh treated his insomnia with "a very strong dose of camphor in my pillow and mattress."

• What about sex before going to sleep? Here is what *Vogue* magazine has to say: "Many people believe that orgasm is a highly potent sedative. This may be true for some individuals, but not all. Kinsey in his book, *Sexual Behavior of the Human Female*, indicated that the period of relaxation after orgasm lasts only a very short time . . . from four to five minutes. What's more, many couples make love during the day and then go to work, drive cars, play tennis, and engage in other activities which would be unsuccessful or downright dangerous if they were very sleepy."

Nonetheless, most men we asked about it think it does wonders for their sleep.

CHAPTER TEN

SLEEP CENTERS
New Hope For Chronic Insomniacs

Perhaps the most significant and prophetic new development in the field of sleep disorders is the rapid rise of the malady as a bona fide specialty among medical professionals.

Interest in sleep began in earnest only slightly more than a decade ago, when doctors started to use information about sleep as an aid to diagnosing illness. As interest grew, disorders of sleep became, in themselves, the subject of laboratory research. This was made possible largely by the development of sophisticated technology that allowed for the rigorous analysis of sleep. Scientists needed a basic understanding of the normal patterns of sleep to use as a standard. How could they help a person with a problem unless they knew exactly what constituted a normal night's sleep?

As a result of this intensive research, scientists are now able to chart the physiological events that occur during sleep with remarkable accuracy. More has been learned about sleep in the last 15 years than in the entire history of human inquiry.

What began as sleep laboratories, where pure research was emphasized, soon turned into sleep *clinics*, where the treatment of patients was the main concern. It happened spontaneously four or five years ago. The researchers were the ones who knew sleep best, and, being doctors and psychiatrists themselves, they were naturally the ones to whom other doctors sent patients with sleep problems.

"The first real center was established in California, at Stanford University," explains Dr. Elliot Weitzman, director of the second one in New York's Montefiore Hospital. "Dr. William Dement was clearly the pioneer. He established a clinic where patients would come. But very quickly a number of us who had been involved in the field of sleep research and the general, scientific issues, were asked to see patients.

"I had been doing a lot of research and had published a lot, and, being a neurologist, I would be referred patients. I would see them just as individuals. I never wanted to start a clinic because it would interfere with other work. Then, after Dement got started, and my own interests moved in that direction, we started one. Theirs and ours are the two largest centers in the United States."

Sleep research exploded in a burst of new information, which has undergone a period of consolidation and dissemination to the rest of the medical community. Now this infant science is leaning more toward clinical application than pure research. The priority now seems to be helping people— something that should make insomniacs rejoice.

With more and more individuals beginning to specialize in the treatment of sleep problems, the need for quality control became evident. The Association of Sleep Disorder Centers was established in Cincinnati to provide a sort of central clearinghouse of knowledge. The Association, composed of leading specialists from all over the country, is attempting to set rigorous standards and certification requirements for sleep centers (the name "center" is preferred to "clinic" or "laboratory"). Committees visit all applicants to inspect and analyze their equipment and procedures.

The goal is to have perhaps two dozen fully equipped centers in major population areas, with a "second tier" of units—less elaborately appointed—spread out across the country. At the more numerous, smaller facilities, patients will be diagnosed, screened, and referred to the appropriate center, if necessary.

The certified sleep centers, we learned from Dr. Charles Pollack, co-director at Montefiore, are seen as regional resources for a given population. They must be associated with a major medical center, with all the important disciplines tied into it in a formal, participatory way. The centers must have the ability to reach out to specialists—internists, neurologists, ear-nose-throat experts, psychiatrists, cardiologists, and so forth. A physician must be retained in a central, active role.

Every center must be equipped with the elaborate technology needed to perform *polysomnograms*—the night-long recordings of physiological variables that we will describe shortly; these are felt to be indispensible—the key to the scientific diagnosis of sleep disorders. Technical standards are now being set for this new procedure, and for the practical requirements for performing it—proper rooms, privacy, emergency care, and other factors must be available.

Training standards are also being established for the technicians who are responsible for the maintenance of the machines and the monitoring of the all-night sessions. Importantly, standards are also being set for the training of those who interpret the complicated recordings. They will be called polysomnographers, and will be taken exclusively from the ranks of M.D. s and psychologists with PhD s.

While the emphasis at these centers will clearly be to deliver high quality medical care, research will be encouraged as well—but only with the patients' explicit consent, and in such a way that it does not interfere with treatment. According to Dr. Pollack, the Association wants to distinguish clearly between laboratories, where experimentation is the priority, and the treatment-oriented centers. Research needs will be met as a matter of course. Each center will keep statistical data (a sleep disorders journal is planned), and in this way the knowledge acquired in the course of treating patients will be shared. Our understanding of sleep disorders, and our ability to treat them, should, as a result, increase geometrically in the next decade.

As of this writing there are five certified centers—those at Stanford, Montefiore (New York), Pittsburgh, Houston, and Columbus, Ohio. Cincinnati's center, Dr. Pollack predicted, will probably be certified by the time you read this.

It should be noted that treatment by specialists is not restricted to those centers that have the sophistication necessary for certification by the Association. Excellent care is available at sleep clinics with less elaborate facilities, headed by highly-qualified and well-informed individuals. The best of these resources, and the certified centers, are listed in the Appendix.

Top Level Panel Discussion on Sleep

In order to give you a better understanding of the centers and clinics, we interviewed several of the leading figures in the field, and one of us actually went through all the procedures as a patient.

First, the interviews. These were actually conducted on separate occasions. with one interviewee at a time. We edited the interviews and put them together to read as though it were a panel discussion. The participants:

–Dr. Ernest Hartmann, director of the Sleep Clinic at Boston State Hospital, Boston, Massachusetts.

–Dr. Peter Hauri, Director of the Sleep Clinic at Dartmouth Medical School, Hanover, New Hampshire.

–Dr. Charles Pollack, co-director of the Sleep-Wake Disorders Unit, Montefiore Hospital, Bronx, New York.

–Dr. Quentin R. Regestein, director of the Sleep Clinic at Peter Bent Brigham Hospital, Boston, Massachusetts.

–Dr. Elliot D. Weitzman, director of the center at Montefiore.

Question: Are the sleep clinics doing pretty much the same work or are there differences?

Weitzman: There are significant differences in our centers, depending on the orientation of each. Ours arose primarily out of the department of neurology. We have a strong psychiatric input, but our interests are broad, and cover a wide range of disorders. Other clinics, like Dr. Hartmann's and Dr. Kales', are more concerned with psychiatric aspects of sleep disorders than we are.

Pollack: We started with the idea of a multidisciplinary approach, with the active collaboration of neurology and psychiatry, to make it as nonbiased as possible. We also have active participation by clinical psychologists. We've retained that orientation for 2½ years. Each center tends to have a different emphasis—it will have its own local character and qualities, depending on who the founder was and what their interests are. We feel this fosters creative and imaginative treatment. At the same time, there is a need for uniform national standards—a center will meet certain stringent requirements, and also apply what it does best.

Weitzman: What sets the differences is, I think, the referral base from which the patients come. If your primary interest is in psychiatric issues, you'll get patients referred to you with those problems. If your primary interest is in narcolepsy, you'll get patients referred with that problem. You tend to look at things according to your own experience.

Question: What percentage of your patients have insomnia?

Pollack: In our center, about 40 percent are insomnia complaints. The majority have excessive daytime sleepiness. They are most often in the categories of narcolepsy and apnea.

Weitzman: Apnea is of particular interest in our center. We didn't decide to study that. The patients just started to come, and once you have some success, it becomes known and the patients come to you. We see eight or ten new patients a week. With the follow-up, that's a lot of patients. We're three months behind. Patients have to wait.

Question: What do you do when a patient comes to you with insomnia?

Weitzman: First of all, we do not look upon insomnia as a disease or a pathology. It is a complaint. It's like a headache, a backache, or a pain in the right hand, or whatever. It's a complaint. It's not an entity in that sense.

Hartmann: I think of insomnia as a symptom, not as a disease. It is not an illness for which the sleeping pill is the cure. Especially in severe cases, you don't want to just treat the symptom. It's like giving a person an aspirin to lower a fever instead of finding the cause. First, we have to determine what is producing the insomnia; is it from something simple, like jet lag? Or working too hard? Or is there something more complicated going on?

Pollack: There is no "typical insomniac." There are many forms of it. All you can really say is it is an inability to fall asleep or stay asleep. The categories of diagnosis are fuzzier than we'd like them to be. It is hard to categorize, but we can treat it even without exact diagnosis.

Weitzman: We have a few basic diagnostic categories: Severe emotional depression—that's a sizeable number of patients. If you treat their depression, the insomnia will improve. Another category is those with nocturnal myoclonus, abnormal twitching of the legs during sleep, and for which we have no known cure. A third category is those patients who have so-called "drug-dependency insomnia." A fourth is those who have a circadian rhythm disturbance, a phase shift of their innate sleep-wake cycle that they interpret as insomnia.

Aging is another factor. My hypothesis is that aging affects a variety of things, including the organization of circadian rhythms. Older people are troubled with awakenings at night, and take little naps during the day. Then there are those with medical problems that disturb sleep—gastrointestinal pain, pain in the feet or back, and so forth. And finally, a whole group of patients with whom we don't know what the cause is.

Hartmann: Some people really produce the whole problem by worrying. The sleep problem may be mild, but they make it much worse by worrying. Another bad mistake, of course, is that people keep taking sleeping pills. Then, when they stop, their sleep is disturbed and they think they need to keep taking more pills.

Hauri: At our clinic, patients undergo a three-day evaluation before any sort of treatment is initiated. There are extensive interviews, physicial examinations, and three nights on the EEG machines to analyze exactly what the sleep pattern is, objectively. We specialize in treating insomnia behaviorally, in helping people overcome sleep-damaging habits.

Regestein: First, I interview them for about an hour to determine exactly what the problem is, what type of insomnia they have, how often it occurs, when it started, what their sleep habits are, and whether they use any drugs, stimulants or sleeping pills. Even nose drops or aspirin can affect sleep.

I ask them extensive questions about their physical health, headaches, eye problems (such as blurring), family health history—whether there are any relatives with sleep disorders. At this point I have enough rapport with the patient to ask more personal questions about his life, his job, his marriage.

If I can't make any conclusions about the cause of the patient's insomnia at this point, I ask him to come back for another interview. I send the patient home with homework—to keep a chart of his sleep patterns, comments on his moods during the day.

I design my treatment according to the person's behavioral history. If my suggestions don't work, then we try the sleep lab to see if perhaps there is anything like myoclonic jerks or some other less obvious answer to the problem.

[Author's note: the intake procedures are fairly standard; we describe them in detail when we recount a visit to a sleep center.]

Question: When is it appropriate to go to a clinic?

Pollack: A physician should seriously consider referral when insomnia is chronic. Say, for several months. Or, when a patient is not responding to available treatments, or when the situation is complicated by some peculiar symptom that the local physician doesn't understand.

Sleep centers should be facilities of almost last resort. The level of expertise there is higher than in the general medical community. Most doctors jump to medication, or to multiple medication if one doesn't work.

Weitzman: People should go to a clinic if they have excessive sleepiness during the day, particularly if they snore heavily. Snoring is the hallmark of sleep apnea. Also, if they have symptoms of narcolepsy or catalepsy, which are lifelong diseases, it's important to have a proper diagnosis made.

Hauri: In many cases, self-diagnosis is possible. But if your problem is still unsolved, then talk to someone who knows all about sleep disorders. Sometimes the problem can be very subtle and of a totally unsuspected nature.

If you are trying to choose a sleep laboratory for diagnosis and treatment, check with the Association of Sleep Disorder Centers.

Hartmann: Self-diagnosis can be done. You can get some hint of what might be causing your problem by just looking at lists of common causes. There are physical and also psychological reasons which people can become aware of in their own lives.

Ask yourself: Am I always tense? Am I preoccupied with problems? Do my muscles tense up in bed? Do I have trouble letting go? Have I been putting an unusual strain on my system? How are my eating habits?

A fair number of people can cure their own insomnia by regulating their eating habits better, getting more exercise, and just learning how to relax. If you've gotten into the habit of going to bed at a different time every night, then a simple change in this damaging habit can help.

Hauri: With insomniacs who have behaviorally related problems (not physiological ones) there are usually three or four factors at work: Some people try too hard to sleep. They have perhaps had a crisis in their lives and had trouble sleeping. Then they started worrying about sleep and started trying too hard, and thus the vicious cycle begins.

Then there are people who are conditioned against their bedroom. One student who couldn't sleep came to me. I asked if he ever slept well. He said yes, on the side of a mountain when he had to be held by ropes so he wouldn't fall while asleep. I understood this to be a totally different situation from his bedroom. The change of environment makes the difference. These people sleep well in the lab. Sleeping on a waterbed or in a hammock or on the floor will often help in this kind of case.

We use something called stimulus control training, developed by Dr. Richard Bootzin. I tell them to try sleeping in the living room. I explain to them that their problem is an association of the bed with frustration. I emphasize that they should never lie in bed awake, that they should go to bed only when tired and ready to sleep.

Then there are bad habits of different sorts—diet, irregularity, chronic tension, and so on.

Hartmann: I don't believe that everyone should visit a physician. As I see it, there are generally three groups of people who have "normal" sleep difficulties, and do not necessarily need to visit a sleep lab. First, the older people who wake up more during the night and are afraid they are not getting enough sleep. We always tell them, of course, that a normal part of aging is needing less sleep and sleeping lighter.

Then there are the people who suffer from anxiety over an event in their lives, like an up-coming exam, or a personal tragedy. That kind of insomnia usually clears up on its own, and most of the population has experienced it in one form or another.

The third category is the short sleepers, the ones who sleep maybe five hours and feel that they don't sleep enough since their mothers always told them to get eight hours. These are short sleepers, they're not insomniacs. There's really no reason they should even worry about their sleep.

But, if it's a severe insomnia of long standing, I do think a visit to the physician can help to determine whether the problem is perhaps of physiological origin—something glandular perhaps—or something else that is not obvious. If the person feels that the problem is really serious and is interfering with his life, then he would benefit from a visit to a sleep clinic or physician. The doctor can then isolate the cause.

The test of whether you should visit a sleep lab is your daytime functioning and daytime mood.

Weitzman: If the patient is a chronic insomniac, and it's not something that just comes and goes, he should certainly see a physician. If he is not satisfied, if it doesn't solve the problem, then he should be seen in a clinic. The sleeplessness should bother him. It should interfere with his functioning. Then it's time to visit a clinic.

Question: Coming to a sleep center is an expensive proposition, isn't it?

[Note: The fee schedule at Montefiore, a typical one, is $150 for initial evaluation—medical history, general and neurological examinations, analysis of sleep log, psychological tests, and reviews by the staff—; and, according to the patient's needs, a short polysomnogram, $75, eight-hour polysomnogram, $200, each additional polysomnogram, $100, psychiatric consultation, $100, and additional fees depending on the extent of follow-up needs.]

Weitzman: Yes, it's relatively expensive. But, we find that it's much less than the patient paid before being taken care of, not only for pills, but wrong diagnoses, or inadequate therapy—I mean, thousands of dollars. This is particularly true of the narcolepsy group. We did an informal survey of our patients and found that it's about ten years from the onset of symptoms before the proper diagnosis is made. Generally, something like eight or ten doctors have been seen before then.

I think the actual benefit to patients is significantly greater than the cost involved, considering the cost of the alternatives. The other point is, I know of no sleep clinic that makes money. They lose money. We're losing money all the time—it's expensive to run the centers.

Question: Do insurance policies cover treatment in a sleep center?

Weitzman: Yes, if it's a severe enough problem. Patients don't come to us with minor problems. It's really the hard-core, serious, chronic problems that come. They've usually seen many doctors. The insurance companies will pay for that. The problem is whether the insurance company will pay for the polysomnogram recording. That's where the problem comes in. It depends on the kind of insurance the person is carrying. Most people don't have good insurance, and they are not covered for that kind of test.

It's a laboratory test, and there are all kinds of complicated ways that policies read regarding it. Blue Cross has agreed, and they're paying for these tests.

Question: Is the polysomnogram indispensible?

Weitzman: In most cases. In some cases, it's obvious that we don't have to do it. Occasionally, we have a patient with, say, a severe major psychosis—severely depressed, suicidal. We're not going to fool around. We immediately get him to the proper care. We've also had patients who have been clear, classic narcoleptics. You just take their history and you know.

Question: What percentage of patients do the centers actually cure?

Hartmann: I'm an optimist. I would say at least 75 or 85 percent can be helped significantly.

Hauri: We won't come up with any magical solutions. What we will come up with is, very likely, a reasonable hypothesis about what might be causing the sleep disturbance ... I mean, whether it is neurological in origin, or secondary to some medical or psychological problem, or something else. And this educated guess will be followed by a list of several recommendations about what that person might then do. Usually—in about 75 to 80 percent of our cases—one of these recommendations will work well, and we'll get a cure. The person will be able to sleep much better."

Regestein: 90 percent of the depressed individuals who come to us with sleep problems are helped. They are usually fairly mild insomniacs and respond well to encouragement and practical suggestions. Sixty or 70 percent of the tense people who come here are able to learn to relax (through progressive relaxation, or meditation, or whatever we find works for them). Once they learn how to let go, their insomnia usually clears up quite dramatically.

The most difficult patients are the ones we call the "restless youth syndromes." These are the people who are usually in the third decade of life, unemployed, with very bad life-styles. They stay up late, have little energy because of poor eating and perhaps drinking or drug-taking, feel no purpose in life and are generally inactive and unmotivated. They are disorganized, estranged, brought up in a chaotic family, often drifting. Their meals are irregular and they get no exercise.

With these people we emphasize regularity in their habits and mealtimes; we try to help their bodies to return to the ebb and flow of normal physiology. But the success rate with these people is only about 15 percent.

Question: Do patients tend to expect too much?

Pollack: The patients' expectations are usually too high. They expect a magical cure. You introduce something new and people with problems think, Eureka! the cure has been found. There is too much emphasis in medicine on breakthrough miracles. There has been a sad underutilization of prevention—too much orientation toward intervention—so people expect instant cures. Often they don't have the willingness to do anything from their side.

Sometimes, however, we have to *raise* the patient's expectations. Patients may not believe they can be helped.

It is difficult to know the actual success rate. You're

dealing with long-term, complex problems with many causes. Our goal is to head the patient in the right direction. We're satisfied when we know that the patient has done certain things and is on the road to taking other steps. You need one or two years to really assess over-all results and our center is only two years old.

I feel that most patients can be and are helped to some extent. Some can't be helped by us, and I don't know if anyone can help them. With serious psychosis, for example, our treatment is just as limited as the treatment of psychosis always is.

Question: Do you do a follow-up on the patients?

Hauri: There is a nine-month follow-up. I write to the referring physician and to the patient. Three out of four— almost 80 percent—say that the clinic was helpful. They sleep much better. Most of the patients say it was worth the $300. I also compare sleep logs that the patients keep nine months after they finished treatment. Seventy percent of the time their sleep patterns look much better.

Pollack: We tend to have close follow-up here. It's primarily a referral facility—we diagnose and refer, usually back to the patient's physician. Finding a suitable psychiatrist is difficult. We work with the psychiatrist or physician and we follow up the patient jointly, especially if medication is being used.

Question: Can you say something about the use of sleeping pills?

Hartmann: Sleeping pills are totally unspecific in their effects on the body. They have basically nothing to do with what we know about sleep. They will never cure insomnia, and should not be used. They are in fact quite dangerous. What you're really taking is a death pill or a coma pill, an anesthetic in a small dose.

Question: What if a person went to a physician who prescribed sleeping pills. What would your advice be?

Weitzman: It depends on the situation. If he says, well, now you're going to have to take this medication from now on, or if one medication doesn't work and the doctor says, take more of this, I would say that he should stop.

In some cases, with short-term acute problems of anxiety—real problems—we may prescribe drugs. On a short-term basis. I recommend Dalmane, which is useful temporarily. More recently, there's been some work that suggests that l-tryptophan, which is really not a drug, works well. It's interesting, if you want to get the drug companies to make it, you've got to have a real drug that harms you. But you can get tryptophan now in health food stores.

Question: Have you prescribed diets for your patients?

Hartmann: Certainly, regular meals, but specifics of diet are a little trickier. I think there are certain substances that can help sleep, and certainly certain vitamin deficiencies such as niacin deficiency that can cause insomnia. We've found that Mexicans particularly suffer from insomnia-causing deficiencies since their diets consist largely of corn products which are devoid of niacin and tryptophan.

I have a sense that getting larger amounts of various vitamins and minerals is very important, but it's surprising how little is really known in this area. I've had a few people who have helped their insomnia by taking magnesium salts. Perhaps the reason for this is the important balance between magnesium and calcium.

Weitzman: There really should be some studies of this. There have not been really good studies, because in order to do them, somebody has to pay for them. Drug companies won't, because they can't make any money on it. The companies that are making things like tryptophan are little companies. They're not about to do research. The FDA is not authorized to do research. They have a minimal budget, and nothing for research. The NIH might do it if somebody came in with a big grant, so it's possible.

Question: What do you foresee for the future?

Weitzman: The whole issue of sleep disorders now, and probably for many years to come, is a nosological one—how do you organize your knowledge? How do you categorize entities? How do you separate A from B? It's a new clinical field.

We want to study patients in our isolation environment and see how they differ from the normal population in their age group. If a patient is a chronic insomniac, we will put him in an environment where he has no clues of time and has no pressure—nothing, totally isolated. Will he establish a good sleep-wake cycle? Will he do as any normal person would? Or, will he continue to have insomnia?

We will be isolating environmental factors, and many other things. We will measure everything—their sleep, their body temperature, their hormones. It's a very elaborate study, and very carefully done. We will then be able to determine what are the laws that structure our sleep-wake cycle. We will learn what the relationship is between variables—how the temperature moves in relation to the sleep stage pattern, and other factors. Do they go together? Is one controlling in some way?

Then we can manipulate, shift sleep, and see what moves and what doesn't. It's a method of studying the relationship among various measurable properties without producing a sleep deprivation.

We've run these experiments with people for two to three weeks. We even had one person for 3½ months. They get a lot done—no telephone, nobody bothering you.

Pollack: There will be enormous progress in the next decade. For one thing, the role of sleep centers will change. Local doctors will know more about sleep disorders and will treat them locally. The referrals to the centers will then be razor sharp.

There will never be *a* single cure. That dream is based on a misconception of insomnia. Certain kinds of insomnia will be helped. We are sharpening our diagnostic acumen; we will have sharply defined categories, and therefore better treatment. That has improved markedly already.

We will have a better understanding of circadian cycles. We will gain a better understanding of how psychological symptoms relate to sleep problems. The relationship is complex, and it may improve our understanding of psychosomatic illness in general. We will also know more about the reverse—how fluctuations in the sleep-wake cycle affect daytime behavior.

One of the most important breakthroughs will be the development of outpatient measures—physiological recordings taken at home. This has vast implications for diagnosis, treatment, and research. For certain disorders, longer recordings are needed than the few days we can do here. The patient will do it in his own bedroom. The cost will go down and the capacity for the amount of recordings will go up. Already there are devices for measuring any biological activity that can be converted into electrical impulses, with the exception of brain waves. We have a device that can measure body temperature every two minutes for a week. There will be ramifications for all of medicine.

Sleeping and waking are all-pervasive. The cycle affects all of life. It is so basic and fundamental that, by knowing more about it, we will know a lot about human behavior that we don't know now.

With sleeping and waking, we're really talking about the fabric of time, and therefore the fabric of existence—how life is structured by human beings. It may lead to a reassessment of the nature of existence.

A Visit To A Sleep Center

The Sleep-Wake Disorders Unit at Montefiore Hospital is a basement suite in a building that neighbors the main hospital. On entering I was startled by the color of the walls—bright, bold yellow with a touch of orange hue. Hardly the subdued, somnolent color I had expected in a place meant to help people sleep. It was, during the day, a bustling place.

In the outer office, surrounded by files and reference shelves, with the constant clatter of a typewriter and the intermittent ring of the telephone, I filled out forms consisting of routine questions about my personal life and my reasons for being there.

Having filled out my forms, I wandered through the rest of the place while waiting for my interview with Dr. Charles Pollack, co-director of the center. Lining a short corridor were comfortable offices and examination rooms. Then, in the rear, I came to a central control room flanked by three pristine, but comfortable, bedrooms. To a layman like me, the control panels looked as awesome as the interior of a space craft—tall, gray units with hundreds of buttons, dials, levers, knobs, and bulbs.

Those were the polygraph machines to which the sleeping patients are attached, via wires and electrodes. Each of their various physiological changes is converted into electrical impulses and recorded on sheets of paper that unwind from a pile and roll under the feathery pens that trace the wavy lines, as though guided by unseen hands. It seemed simultaneously like a testament to the wonders of the human intellect, and a thoroughly ludicrous game—something as fundamental as sleep reduced to lines and numbers!

My interview with Dr. Pollack lasted an hour. A neurologist, he asked me about the history of my sleep problem—when did it first occur? under what circumstances? did any particular event bring it on? what was the exact pattern of a typical night?

He was inquisitive about my family history: did anyone else have insomnia? how was their mental and physical health? He asked about my personal life: relationships, career, money, drugs. He asked about my sleep habits: unusual positions, breathing problems, snoring, kicking, moving around. He asked about how I usually felt during the day, and, of course, he wanted my medical history.

Before passing me on to the psychologist, Dr. Arthur Spielman, Dr. Pollack pointed out that I was wearing two hats. I was there as a patient and also as a reporter; the dual role might influence my treatment and my impressions. It was a point well taken, and it should be marked by the reader.

Dr. Spielman's interview began much like Dr. Pollack's, but he soon began digging more deeply into my psychic underbrush. His first question was, "Why are you here?" He wanted to know what runs through my mind when I lie awake at night. He probed for obsessions, compulsions, fears, and underlying patterns that might indicate neuroses. At least that's what I thought he was doing.

Where the physician seemed to be looking for medical causes, the psychologist (he was not a psychiatrist, and therefore did not have an M.D.) seemed to be looking for events—real or imagined, outer or inner—that might trigger sufficient anxiety, or sufficient depression, to keep me awake.

Without being offensive, he inquired about basic personal feelings, and my perceptions of my career, my love life, my relationships, my health, my self.

Afterward, I sat at a desk in the bedroom where, two

months later, I would spend a night. I filled out a battery of psychological tests: personality tests, interest and preference tests, self-evaluative questionnaires, an inventory of recent life changes, questionnaires about sleep habits and patterns and levels of daytime alertness, and the Minnesota Multiphasic Personality Inventory, perhaps the most highly regarded of the tests that purport to measure patterns of neurosis and psychosis.

It was, I admit, so tedious I rushed through quickly and requested permission to take some tests home with me. It was partially granted. But the questionnaires themselves—regardless of what they told the doctors—were valuable. They made me reflect upon questions I needed to ask myself.

Back to Dr. Pollack. He joined me in an austere examination room with a stethoscope and little black bag in hand. He gave me a complete physical. Then, turning to his specialty, he put me through some fascinating paces—literally.

First, I paced up and down the room. Then I paced on my heels, then my toes, then as though on a tightrope. I hopped in place on each foot. Then, both seated and supine, I had to react quickly to a rapid succession of stimuli—tuning forks, flashlights and Dr. Pollack's fingers. The stimuli came at me from all angles in varying degrees of intensity. I had to react quickly: where did I touch you? how many fingers did I hold up? what do you see? can you hear this?

It was all designed to identify possible defects in the central nervous system. I had a great time, and I passed with flying colors—and flying sounds and flying taps as well.

A urine specimen, a blood test, and a blood pressure test later, my 4½-hour evaluation was almost over. I was dressed and back in Dr. Pollack's office. He looked over my sleep log, which I had been asked to keep for two weeks prior to my visit.

I was given an appointment for my all-night polysomnogram for two months later. Until then, Dr. Pollack advised, I was to establish a precise bedtime and a precise waking-up time. I was to stick to that routine conscientiously. I groaned. As a writer, I had been able to sleep and wake according to my own moods and needs. I liked having that freedom, and was partially convinced that it was necessary for my craft. I did not like the idea of stopping an activity just because the clock said I should. Suppose I wasn't tired?

Moreover, I didn't like waking up to alarms. My insomnia deprived me of enough sound sleep, I thought, why should I lose any more? I recalled a line from a Marx brothers' movie. "Don't wake him," says Chico to Groucho, "he's got insomnia and he's trying to sleep it off." What was even worse was the prospect of giving up my afternoon naps, a luxury that had long since become a frequent necessity.

Dr. Pollack, with admirable patience, explained that the regimen was a temporary one. He emphasized the importance of regularity in maintaining normal sleep. It was especially important for someone like me, he said, whose sleep time varied as much as three to four hours from one day to the next. He wanted to get a rhythm going before my sleep was recorded in the lab. Then he would be better able to evaluate my condition. He would have a clearer picture of the patterns my body naturally assumed, when free of arbitrary impositions. Once the pattern was known, he said, and I had had my evaluation, I could be more flexible.

Somewhat relieved, I attempted to bargain on the naps. He said I should either eliminate them or take them every day at the same time. The important thing was to set a pattern and stick to it. Most people are unable to find the time for a nap, given customary social and vocational necessities, and opt for eliminating them. Grateful, I chose to keep them.

At the time of that initial evaluation, my insomnia had become only an erratic problem, closely correlated with the level of stress in my life, and, I believe, with my eating and exercising patterns. It was not terribly severe. *I would not have gone to a sleep center if I had not been a reporter*. I emphasize that, because my opinions and experience were undoubtedly influenced by that fact. I was not—neither in motivation nor symptoms—a typical patient. Nonetheless, we felt that this record was revealing, and would provide the reader with a firsthand account of sleep centers from the patient's viewpoint, the first such report to appear in print, we believe.

By the time my overnight recording was done, I was even more atypical. I still awakened prematurely, but not as often, and not as annoyingly as I once had. I attribute the change to several factors: the use of some of the procedures discussed earlier (notably TM, exercise, and diet); to the sophistication I'd acquired while researching this book (I no longer would fret over premature awakenings. Instead, I would do a breathing or relaxation technique, or eat some protein, and just not worry. Usually, I fell asleep fairly quickly. When I did not, I just got up and started my day, napping later on if necessary); and, finally, to my adherence (I'll admit to more cheating than Dr. Pollack would have liked) to regular sleep-wake patterns.

The latter point is an interesting one. It had not been easy for me to adhere to a set pattern. It was, in fact, a major readjustment, and I was not as disciplined as I should have been. But it helped. That help alone might be worth the price to a chronic insomniac. Somehow, even to a patient with a convenient excuse (I'm just in it as a reporter), doctor's orders are doctor's orders. You tend to stick to them.

I arrived for my polysomnogram while another patient was getting ready for bed and a second was being hooked up. I watched as two graduate students who serve as part-time technicians adroitly placed the electrodes on the skin of a heavyset, middle-aged man with a rosy-cheeked smile and an expression of equal parts fascination and apprehension. He told me that it didn't hurt a bit, as had the other patient, a woman in her 70s who had been suffering with insomnia for several years and had tried "everything." She was convinced that her problem was emotional and she did not have much hope that the center could help. I wondered why, feeling that way, she would invest so much money in this procedure.

I asked the technicians questions as they worked on the man, and they were gracious enough to answer in detail. The two electrodes on the man's chin were for making an electromyogram measurement, which indicates body muscle tone, or tension. The electrodes they placed on the corner of the eyes were for measuring rapid eye movement—apparently, as the eyes move, an electric field moves with it, generated from tissue in the retina. The electrodes pick up the changes.

All of the electrodes, by the way, are arranged in pairs. If one falls off during the night, the second serves as a back-up, enabling the technicians to continue the monitoring without disturbing the patient. Also, it should be noted, electrodes are placed *on* the surface of the skin; they are not inserted as if they were needles.

On the forehead, the technicians placed a "ground" to

prevent picking up ambient electromagnetic activity. The patient, hooked up in that way, might otherwise serve as an antenna.

Two electrodes were glued to the top of the scalp to detect brain waves. Electrodes were placed on the upper right of the chest, and on the lower left. These were for the electrocardiogram. Temperature-sensitive devices were taped beneath the mouth and at the entrance of each nostril—these picked up the breath rate (number per minute) and the volume of air taken in. Finally, an electrode was placed on each shin, or, in anatomical jargon, on the "anterior tibia." This shows restlessness, and is vital for detecting nocturnal myoclonus.

This particular patient had several things done that I did not. For one thing, his two EEG electrodes were placed differently—mine were both on top of the head, while his were on top and rear respectively. The second difference was that he had a small microphone placed beneath his nose, to enable the technicians to hear his breathing. The third difference was that he was videotaped. An infrared camera (no lights needed) photographs the patient all night long. The technician watches on a monitor, and can adjust the camera angle from the control room. The screen is split—half shows the sleeping patient, while the other half shows the ongoing readouts from the polysomnogram.

The reason for the differences, I was told, was basically that I had insomnia, while the other man was suspected of having apnea. Thus the need for hearing him breathe, and for watching him. An insomniac's restlessness can be detected without seeing him.

Finally it was my turn to be hooked up. I watched the other patient, wires dangling behind him like reins from a horse's bit, wisps of cotton rising from the electrodes as he carefully stepped toward the bedroom. He was self-conscious and tried not to disturb the wires that ran up the legs of his pajamas. We waved and wished each other a good night's sleep.

In order to make the electrodes adhere to the skin, the technicians rub the site with alcohol, acetone, and sodium chloride. This apparently removes the outer surface of cells and also makes the skin less resistant to current. It did not hurt except on the shins, where, for some reason, it burned

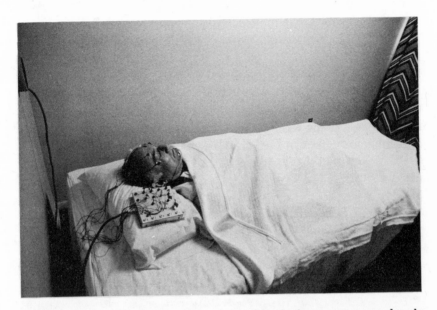

A sleeping patient wears the electrodes and leads that are connected to the polysomnograph machine in the adjoining monitoring area of the Sleep-Wake Disorders Unit. The machine records brain waves, chin muscle tone, eye movement, respiration and heart rate. Depending upon the disorder, diagnosticians also place electrodes on other parts of the body.

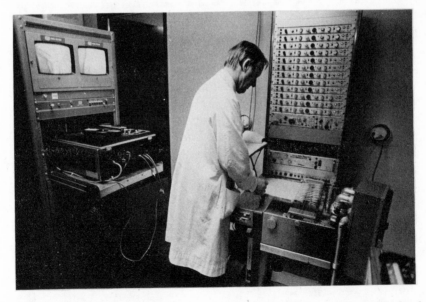

In the Sleep-Wake Disorders Unit at Montefiore Hospital and Medical Center, a technician checks a polysomnogram (a recording of sleep stages) of a patient asleep in an adjacent room. The videotape recorder, at left, monitors and records the patient's body movements.

slightly. The only discomfort I felt came from the obnoxious odor of the acetone. When they applied it anywhere near my nose I was tempted to run out. I could not, of course, because I was already partially wired up.

The electrodes did not hurt, but I was very aware of them. They were like flies that couldn't be shooed away. Eventually, I got used to their presence, as the technicians and the other patients (who were seasoned pros, having done this the night before) had assured me I would. The technicians said that the wires and electrodes rarely interfere with anyone's sleep. In fact, many people sleep unusually well in the lab because they are removed—physically and psychologically—from the environment in which they usually have difficulty. Perhaps there is something self-fulfilling about going someplace to sleep better.

As they hooked me up, I watched the electric pens record the sleep of my two fellow patients. The occasional bursts, I was informed, were the result of legs or chins moving. The man on the TV screen fell asleep quickly. Soon, he snored. We could see when his breathing became obstructed. The screen image corresponded perfectly to certain indexes on the EEG and other read-outs.

When they were finished securing my electrodes, the technicians yanked on the wires to see if they were firmly secured.

My bedroom was pleasant enough, painted a bright yellow. An attractive still life of flowers in a vase hung on the wall. The floors were carpeted, and drapes covered the windows. It would be quiet and absolutely dark.

Before going to bed, I filled out a questionnaire: what time had I awakened that morning? when had I eaten? was the day unusual in any way? how did I feel? what did I expect to happen that night with respect to my sleep?

I climbed into a firm, but unusually high and somewhat narrow bed. The technician hooked up my dangling wires to a box on the corner of the bed. He strapped a beltlike gadget around my waist—loosely, I hardly noticed it. It was a "thoracoabdominal gauge" that measures breathing by detecting the motion of the diaphragm.

As I got into bed, I caught a glimpse of myself in the mirror. I looked as though I belonged next door in the emergency ward. The tape used to hold the electrodes in place looked like bandages, and the wires, innocent as they were, had an ominous look about them. Making the pictorial image worse were the wisps of cotton that emanated from the electrodes. The technicians daub each area with cotton to prevent the glue from sticking to the sheets.

Despite the image in the mirror, I felt quite comfortable. My facial movements were slightly limited, but I soon got used to that. I could tell that my usual sleep positions and movements would not be significantly hampered. I was tired, and more than ready to close my eyes. Ironically, the procedures kept me up past the bedtime that I had established on the doctors' recommendation.

Then, after I had said goodnight and the lights had been turned off, we encountered a technical difficulty. They had placed the leg electrodes too near a vein and were picking up a pulse beat. It took them five or ten minutes to replace the electrodes, and then another few minutes to readjust the device that recorded my mouth breathing. I was annoyed.

My sleep was typical. I fell asleep in what I estimated to be ten minutes but which I later found out was three. I missed my special, cigar-shaped pillow, and was sorry I had not brought it along. At times during the night when I awakened briefly, I could not adjust to the ordinary-style pillow. I was also aware of the wires at those times, and somewhat annoyed by them. But those disturbances were trivial.

At about 4:30, I awakened, restless, tense in the legs, unable to get back to sleep. It was my typical awakening, and in a sense I was glad it had occurred that particular night so the doctors would have something pathological to see. It was eerie in the strange, pitch-black room. Suddenly, I heard a sound that made it even more eerie: a loud roar, as of wind rushing through a tunnel. It repeated itself every few seconds. Finally, I realized what it was. The patient with sleep apnea was snoring and the microphone was blasting the sound into the control room.

I rapped on the wall and called for the all-night technician, a young man named Jerry who had come on at midnight. Jerry promised to lower the sound of the patient's breathing, and he unhooked me so that I might go to the bathroom. It is hard to convey how weird it felt to stagger in a strange place holding a bunch of wires over my shoulder.

When I returned to bed, Jerry plugged me in again. I could not get back to sleep. I was quite restless. I lay there listening to the now-subdued sound of the man snoring, for about ten minutes. Then I propped myself up in bed as far as I could without straining the wires, and practiced TM. Sometime later, more relaxed, I lay down and slept.

I awakened at 7:30, having had an erratic sleep after my trip to the bathroom. I was slightly more groggy than I usually am after a night like that. I showered, finally free of the wires and electrodes, and then Jerry had me fill out a questionnaire. It asked questions about my experiences during the night.

That was it. The stack of paper on which my sleep pattern was indelibly recorded was then sent to a computer, which printed out a summary of my sleep. That is stored for posterity on magnetic tape.

Mr. MacGregor, a cheerful man with a charming Scots accent, analyzed the data for quantitative content—how much time spent in each stage of sleep, number of awakenings, and so on. His analysis was then sent to Dr. Pollack for qualitative interpretation—here some judgement is involved, as the doctor looks for subtle signs of abnormalities. Dr. Pollack conferred with Dr. Speilman, and then made the group's recommendations known to me in a private meeting.

I met with Dr. Pollack less than a week after my night at the center. My own estimates and expectations jibed closely with the polysomnogram data, something that I gathered was not always the case. (I was nonetheless surprised to find that it had taken me half an hour to fall asleep after my trip to the bathroom; I had estimated an hour.) The closeness of my approximation to the actual pattern indicated to the doctors that I was not overly anxious about my insomnia—I was neither overdramatizing it, nor underestimating it.

I did, indeed, have numerous awakenings. Most of them were brief—about 20 seconds—and not of much consequence. The proportion of time spent in each stage of sleep was normal—that had not been disturbed by the awakenings, as it sometimes is. However, I spent too much of the total time awake—15 percent. This was not normal.

In addition, there was one qualitative abnormality: sleep spindles, which ordinarily only occur during Stages II and III of sleep, were occurring in the REM stage with me. It was a relatively mild disorganization of EEG, but it was indicative, Dr. Pollack said, of a chronic disturbance. Sleep spindles take time to develop.

There were no abnormal physiological occurrences, such as apnea or myoclonus, and the arousals did not take place from the REM stage. That indicated to the doctors that my sleep mechanism was intact. "We're dealing with normal machinery," Dr. Pollack said.

My pattern was not unusual, apparently. It was close in style to that seen in depressed patients. "But you are not depressed," the doctor quickly assured me. "The pattern indicates excessive arousal processes during sleep. And that is consistent with your personality. You tend to be somewhat self-critical, somewhat compulsive, easily agitated. You ruminate a lot, and worry too much."

He was certainly right. I reflected that my sleep problems tend to occur at times when those personality traits are unusually dominant, due to circumstances that create stress.

Dr. Pollack explained that thinking processes continue during sleep—it is not a time of complete inertia, but a continuation of psychological processes that occur during wakefulness.

He reassured me that there was nothing pathological about my sleep pattern, strictly speaking. It was "mild insomnia." As for treatment, he and Dr. Spielman agreed that I should avoid sleeping pills at all costs, since, in their estimation, my personality was the type that might abuse them. They might have been right about that had it not been for my recent education about the evils of sleeping pills.

Dr. Pollack admonished me, mildly and good-naturedly, about pushing myself too hard and worrying too much. "Obsessiveness can be useful," he said. "It can lead to success. But it can also be damaging. It's a trade-off."

Neither he nor Dr. Spielman felt it necessary to make any specific clinical recommendation, such as psychotherapy. In light of the mildness of my case, and my relative sophistication about sleep and insomnia, they simply left it up to me to adjust my personality and behavior. They were satisfied that I had already begun taking steps to help myself.

The one thing Dr. Pollack was adamant about was the need to stick to a regular pattern of sleeping and waking times. "It's not that we're against spontaneity or individuality," he explained, "It's just that regularity will help. It's a trade-off. If awakening at night bothers you, then you might have to give up something in order to eliminate the problem."

I was happy to have had the opportunity to go through the clinic, not only for its journalistic value, but for my own understanding of my sleep problem. There was something oddly reassuring about seeing all those wavy lines on a piece of paper. Now I knew exactly what my situation was, and I had the experts' evaluation of its cause. I was no longer burdened with having to contemplate my own conjectures and speculations. The mystery—and therefore the possibility of misinterpretation or self-delusion—was removed.

Dr. Hauri of Dartmouth expressed it well: "Very often they [the patients] arrive here believing they've got a condition far more serious than they actually have. And so they do find some comfort in knowing something more specific about what's really going on."

It can work the other way too. Some patients will make light of their problem to avoid having to do something about it. They hope, when they visit the clinic, that the doctors will conclude that they are normal, or that the doctors will provide them with a miracle cure. Often, they are thrust into the awareness that their sleep problems are their own responsibility. A visit to a clinic might be the impetus they need finally to act. In my case, I was now prepared to take more seriously advice that I'd heard—and had given myself—many times before.

Conclusion

The sleep centers, and the accompanying sophistication about sleep that is developing, signal a new era in human knowledge. All insomniacs—mild and severe—should rejoice in this development. While it is apparent that only the very severe insomniacs need go to a sleep center for treatment, every person with sleep difficulties will ultimately benefit from the centers. For one thing, even now, an individual can gain a great deal from existing sleep clinics by way of expert diagnosis, if the price is within reach. Soon, however, sophisticated diagnostic apparatus will find its way into local doctors' offices, or "second tier" diagnostic clinics, causing the cost to plummet. More important, perhaps, for the average insomniac, will be the spread of information that will ensue as findings become known to the nonspecialists in the medical community and to the public. Treating insomnia, which is often hit or miss, is on the way to becoming more precise.

We can only encourage the trend that has begun; more and more clinics are needed, and more and more research is vital. We hope that funding agencies, both private and public, will see fit to finance sleep research. Few problems are as pandemic as insomnia, and few are as symptomatic of general mental and physical maladies. As Dr. Pollack said earlier, sleep research could shed light on a wide variety of issues that touch the very core of human life.

We were comforted and encouraged by our encounters with sleep specialists. They seemed to us an honorable and dedicated group of professionals, whose sincere efforts are, and will continue to be, an important contribution to human life. The track they are on seems to us both exciting and fruitful.

Yet, we also had a vague uneasiness that we would like to share with them and with the reader. It might be worth questioning whether or not our fascination with gadgetry and technology is somewhat out of proportion. Excessive reliance on expensive, highly complex solutions has, in the past, often created as many problems as it has solved. Often, what seems a perfectly innocent procedure turns out to have unforeseen consequences. Sleeping pills are a good example. We should be extra careful about any device—mechanical or chemical—until all the evidence is in.

In addition, reliance on sophisticated technology seems to make the patient that much more dependent. It requires tremendous expertise to use that equipment—to invent it, build it, maintain it, apply it, evaluate its results. Perhaps attention should also be given to ways in which the patient can become more self-reliant. This would be consistent with the current trend toward increased self-care.

Finally, we would like to see more research done on natural treatments for sleep disorders. It is astonishing, and more than a little disturbing, to see the degree to which nutrition, exercise, meditation, and other self-administering, nontechnical methods are ignored. While very severe disorders may require a great deal more expertise, it seems that, by and large, most insomniacs can be helped considerably with these natural techniques. Data is needed to confirm this.

It seems to us that, while not disregarding the research trends that are already under way (they are vital, it must be emphasized) the scientific community should also address itself to the question: how can we reestablish a symbiotic relationship with nature? Sleep disorders, after all, represent a break from nature. Our top priority should be sealing that break and living once again in harmony with our natural environment. When we do that, we will all sleep better.

BIBLIOGRAPHY

Authors' Note: This bibliography includes all of the most useful books we have consulted in writing this book. The reader will find additional references in the bibliographies of the books listed here. An asterisk * next to the author's name indicates the best books in each category.

1. **Sleep and Insomnia**

    Bauer, W. *All You Need to Know About Insomnia, Sleep and Dreams* (New York: Essandes, 1967)

    Buhler, W. *How to Overcome Sleeplessness* (Los Angeles: Krishna Press, 1973)

    Boulware, Marcus *Snoring: New Answers to an Old Problem* (New York: American Faculty, 1974)

    Crisp, Arthur *Sleep, Nutrition and Mood* (New York: Stonehill, 1976)

    Dement, William *Some Must Watch While Some Must Sleep* (New York: W. H. Freeman, 1974)

    Duncan, A. H. *Everything You Want to Know About Sleep* (New York: Pyramid, 1973)

    Foulkes, David *The Psychology of Sleep* (New York: Scribner's, 1966)

    Gutwirth, Samuel *How to Sleep Well* (New York: Vantage, 1959)

    Hartmann, Ernest L. *The Functions of Sleep* (New Haven: Yale Press, 1973)

    Hill, Wilfred *Good Sleep Without Drugs* (England: Boughton Herald, 1955)

*Jacobson, Edmund *You Can Sleep Well* (Chicago: Whittlesey House, 1938)

Kales, Anthony *Sleep: Physiology and Pathology* (Philadelphia: Lippincott, 1969)

Kelly, Charles *The Natural Way to Healthful Sleep* (New York: Hawthorne, 1961)

Kleitman, Nathaniel *Sleep and Wakefulness* (Chicago: Univ. of Chicago, 1963)

Kohler, M. and Chapelle, J. *101 Recipes for Sound Sleep* (New York: Funk and Wagnalls, 1967)

Laird, D. A. *Sound Ways to Sound Sleep* (New York: McGraw Hill, 1959)

Linde, Shirley *The Sleep Book* (New York: Harper and Row, 1974)

*Luce, Gay and Segal, J. *Insomnia: The Guide for Troubled Sleepers* (New York: Doubleday, 1969)

*Luce, Gay and Segal, J. *Sleep* (New York: Coward-McCann, 1966)

Moolman, Valery *40 Winks at the Drop of a Hat* (New York: Pocket Books, 1973)

Murray, E. J. *Sleep, Dreams and Arousal* (New York: Appleton-Century, 1965)

Oswald, Ian *Sleep* (England: Penguin Books, 1966)

Oswald, Ian *Sleep and Waking* (New York: Elsevier Publishing Co. 1962)

Pai, M. N. *Sleeping Without Pills* (New York: Stein and Day, 1965)

Rosenteur, Phyllis *Morpheus and Me* (New York: Funk and Wagnalls, 1957)

*Rubenstein, Hillary *Insomniacs of the World, Goodnight!* (New York: Random House, 1974)

Scott, Cyril *Good Sleep Without Drugs* (New York: Lust, 1974)

*Steincrohn, Peter *How to Get a Good Night's Sleep* (Chicago: Regnery, 1968)

Thoresen, Carl and Coates, T. *How to Sleep Better* (Englewood Cliffs: Prentice Hall, 1976)

Weitzman, Elliot *Advances in Sleep Research Volumes I and II* (New York: Halsted Press, 1974, 1976)

Webb, Wilse *Sleep: The Gentle Tyrant* (New York: Spectrum, 1975)

2. Sleeping Pills—Drugs

Burack, Richard *The Handbook of Prescription Drugs* (New York: Pantheon, 1967)

Meares, A. *Relief Without Drugs* (New York: Doubleday, 1965)

*Mintz, Morton *The Therapeutic Nightmare* (Boston: Houghton Mifflin, 1965)

3. General Health

Esquire Magazine *The Art of Keeping Fit* (New York: Harper and Brothers, 1952)

Miller, Ethan *Bodymind* (New York: Pinnacle Books, 1974)

*Samuels, Mike *The Well Body Book* (New York: Random House, 1973)

*Selye, Hans *The Stress of Life* (New York: McGraw-Hill, 1956)

4. Chiropractic

*Dintenfass, Julius *Chiropractic: A Modern Way To Health* (New York: Pyramid, 1970)

5. Homeopathy

Kaufman, Martin *Homeopathy in America* (New York: Johns Hopkins, 1971)

6. Hypnosis

Bowers, Kenneth *Hypnosis for the Seriously Curious* (New York: Brooks-Cole, 1976)

Fromm, Erika and Shor, Ronald *Hypnosis: Research Developments and Perspectives* (New York: Aldine, 1972)

7. The Transcendental Meditation Technique

*Bloomfield, Harold *TM: Discovering Inner Energy and Overcoming Stress* (New York: Delacorte, 1975)

*Goldberg, Philip *TM: The Way to Fulfillment* (New York: Holt, 1976)

*McWilliams, Peter *The TM Book* (Los Angeles: Price, Stern, Sloan, 1975)

8. Relaxation Techniques

Jacobson, Edmund *Progressive Relaxation* (Chicago: Whittlesey House, 1938)

Roon, Karin *The New Way to Relax* (New York: Greystone Press, 1949)

Steincrohn, Peter and Lafie, D. *How to Master Your Nerves* (New York: Cowles, 1974)

9. Biofeedback
Karlins, M. and Andrews L. *Biofeedback* (Philadelphia: Lippincott, 1972)

10. Exercise
*Cooper, Kenneth H. *The New Aerobics* (New York: Bantam, 1970)

World Publications *Beginning Running* (P.O. Box 366, Mt. View, CA. 94040)

11. Food and Diet
Bieler, Henry *Food is Your Best Medicine* (New York: Random House, 1965)

*Davis, Adelle *Let's Eat Right to Keep Fit* (New York: Harcourt, Brace Javonovitch, 1954)
   Let's Get Well (New York: Harcourt, Brace and World, 1965)
   Be Happier, Be Healthier (New York: Fawcett, 1962)

*Dufty, William *Sugar Blues* (New York: Warner, 1976)

Fredericks, Carlton *Psycho-Nutrition* (New York: Grosset and Dunlop, 1976)

Hauser, Gaylord *Look Younger and Live Longer* (New York: Farrar, Strauss and Giroux, 1951)

Johnson, Harry *Eat, Drink, Be Merry and Live Longer* (New York: Doubleday, 1965)

Prevention Magazine Editors *The Complete Book of Vitamins* (Emmaus, Pa.: Rodale Press, 1977)

Walker, N. W. *Raw Vegetable Juices* (New York: Pyramid, 1970)

12. Orthomolecular Medicine

Books published by the Huxley Institute (1114 First Avenue, New York, New York 10021)—send for price list:

Consumer's Digest *Megavitamins: A New Hope for The Mentally Ill*

*Cott, Alan *Doctors Speak on the Orthomolecular Approach*

Hoffer, Abram *Supernutrition*

Newbold, A. *How one Psychiatrist Began using Niacin*

*Pauling, Linus *Orthomolecular Psychiatry*

Ross, Harvey *Hypoglycemia*

13. Fasting

Bragg, Paul *The Miracle of Fasting* (California: Health Science Press, 1970)

*Cott, Alan *Fasting: The Ultimate Diet* (New York: Bantam Books, 1975)

Shelton, Herbert *Fasting Can Save Your Life* (Chicago: National Hygiene Press, 1964)

14. Mental and Emotional Health

Carnegie, Dale *How to Stop Worrying and Start Living* (New York: Simon and Schuster, 1948)

Gumpert, Martin *The Anatomy of Happiness* (New York: McGraw-Hill, 1951)

Gutwirth, Samuel *How to Free Yourself from Nervous Tension* (Chicago: Regnery, 1955)

May, Rollo *Man's Search for Himself* (New York: New American Library, 1953)

Miller, Don Ethan *Bodymind* (New York: Pinnacle, 1974)

*Russell, Bertrand *The Conquest of Happiness* (New York: Liveright, 1930)

*Viscott, David S. *Freeing Yourself from Bad Moods* (U.S. Government Printing Office, Washington, D.C. 20402 30¢)
* *The Language of Feelings* (New York: Arbor House, 1975)

Ubell, Earl *How to Save Your Life* (New York: Harcourt, Brace Javonovitch, 1973)

15. Herbs

Ceres, *Herbs to Help you Sleep* (England: Thorsens Publishers, 1972)

Coon, Nelson *Using Plants for Healing* (New York: Heathside Press, 1963)

Kloss, Jethro *Back to Eden* (New York: Beneficial Books, 1971)

*Lust, John *The Herb Book* (New York: Bantam, 1974)

16. Yoga

*Brena, Steven *Yoga and Medicine* (New York: Penguin, 1972)

*Hittleman, Richard *Yoga for Physical Fitness* (New York: Warner, 1967)

Iyengar, B. *Light on Yoga* (New York: Shocken, 1965)

Marx, Ina *Yoga and Common Sense* (New York: Bobbs Merrill, 1970)

17. Massage

*Downing, George *The Massage Book* (New York: Random House, 1972)

  Massage and Meditation (New York: Random House, 1974)

18. Magazine Articles on Sleep

*Diamond, Edwin "Long Day's Journey into the Insomniac's Night" *New York Times Magazine,* p. 31, October 1, 1967

*Trilling, Calvin Reporter at Large: "A Third State of Existence" *The New Yorker,* September 18, 1965

19. Magazine and Journal Articles on Tryptophan

Hartmann, E. L-Tryptophane and Sleep. In *Psychopharmacologia,* 1971, *19,* p. 114

Hartmann, E. The Effect of L-Tryptophane on the Sleep-Dream Cycle in Man. *Psychonomic Science,* 1967, *8,* p. 479

Wyatt, R. L. Engelman, K., Kupfer, D. J., Fram, D. H. Sjoerdsma, A. and Snyder, F. Effects of L-Tryptophane (a natural sedative) on Human Sleep *The Lancet,* 1970, October 24, p. 842

APPENDIX

Sleep-Disorder
Professionals and Sleep Clinics

1. American Association of Sleep Disorder Centers
   University of Cincinnati Sleep Center
   Christian R. Holmes Hospital
   Eden and Bethesda Avenues
   Cincinnati, Ohio 45219

2. Dr. John Beck
   Director
   Southern California Center for Sleep Disorders
   1260 15th Street, Suite 1402
   Santa Monica, California 90404

3. Dr. William C. Dement
   Director
   Stanford University Sleep Disorders Clinic
   Stanford University Medical Center
   Stanford, California 94304

4. Dr. Ernest Hartmann
   Director, New England Sleep Disorders Center
   Boston State Hospital
   591 Morton Street
   Boston, Massachusetts 02124

5. Dr. Peter Hauri
   Director, Sleep Clinic
   Dartmouth Medical School
   Hanover, New Hampshire 03755

6. Dr. Anthony Kales
   Director
   Sleep Research and Treatment Center
   Pennsylvania State University
   Milton S. Hershey Medical Center
   Hershey, Pennsylvania 17033

7. Dr. Allan Hobson
   Director, Laboratory of Neurophysiology
   Massachusetts Mental Health Center
   Harvard Medical School
   25 Shattuck Street
   Boston, Massachusetts 02115

8. Dr. Ismet Karacan
   Director
   Sleep Disorders Clinic
   Baylor College of Medicine
   Houston, Texas 77025

9. Dr. Daniel F. Kripke
   Director
   Sleep Diagnostic Laboratory
   Veterans Administration Hospital
   3350 La Jolla Village Drive
   San Diego, California 92161

10. Dr. Milton Kramer
    Director, Sleep Clinic
    Veterans Administration Hospital
    Cincinnati, Ohio 45220

11. Dr. David Kupfer
    Director
    Sleep Disorders Clinic
    Western Psychiatric Institute and Clinic
    3811 O'Hara Street
    Pittsburgh, Pennsylvania 15261

12. Dr. H. Lemmi
    Mid-South Sleep Disorders Center
    Neurophysiology Lab
    Baptist Memorial Hospital
    Memphis, Tennessee, 38146

13. Dr. William C. Orr
    Director
    Sleep Physiology Laboratory
    Veterans Administration Hospital
    921 N.E. 13th Street
    Oklahoma City, Oklahoma 73104

14. Dr. Quentin R. Regestein
    Director, Sleep Clinic
    Peter Bent Brigham Hospital
    Boston, Mass. 02115

15. Dr. Helmut Schmidt
    Sleep Clinic
    Ohio State University
    Department of Psychiatry
    Columbus, Ohio 43210

16. Dr. Jean-Paul Spire
    Director
    Sleep Disorders Unit
    University of California School of Medicine
    San Francisco, California 94101

17. Dr. Gerald Vogel
    Director of Sleep Laboratory
    Emory University School of Medicine
    Atlanta, Georgia 30322

18. Dr. Elliot D. Weitzman
    Director
    Sleep-Wake Disorders Unit
    Montefiore Hospital and
    Medical Center
    111 East 210th Street
    Bronx, New York 10580

Experts Testify on
Over-the-Counter Sleep Aids

Sumner M. Kalman, M.D.
Professor of Pharmacology
Stanford Medical School

Turning to the sleep-aids, we found three groups of active ingredients, often marketed together or in various combinations. They were bromides, drugs of the atropine-belladonna class, and antihistamines. The bromides we found too dangerous for over-the-counter use because of their tendency to accumulate when used chronically and, by accumulation in the body to pose a serious hazard to health. The use of bromides, although it has dropped out of medical practice in the treatment of sleeplessness or epilepsy, may be carried out safely if bromides are prescribed and if the patients are monitored carefully so that the blood-level of bromides is assessed continuously. The curious way by which bromides work, the displacement of the normal chloride ion in the body by the bromide ion so that a central nervous system depression is achieved, makes the use of these agents totally unsuitable for over-the-counter use. It is not rational for *occasional* use. The atropine-belladonna group of drugs is currently subject to abuse as street drugs. They can cause idiosyncratic effects in patients, even in relatively small doses. They have been used in sub-therapeutic amounts in many preparations which have been marketed. This is probably why people who take them as instructed have not had more toxic reactions. But, because they carry with them certain dangers such as a delusional psychotomimetic reaction in some patients, they should not be used for trivial conditions. The Panel recognized that both

The following statements are excerpted from testimony on over-the-counter sedatives, sleep-aids and stimulant drugs presented before the Senate Select Committee on Small Business, June 14, 1977.

We reproduce only those parts of each statement which deal with sleep inducing drugs.

---

bromides and belladonna alkaloids should not be marketed for casual use as sleep-aids. This led us to the antihistamines. The antihistamines have a central depressant action which is non-specific. We found few careful studies in the submissions given to us by manufacturers, and we had to, as did other panels, look in the scientific literature to find out if there were controlled studies where antihistamines had been given alone. We found evidence that higher doses, not the doses usually used in OTC preparations, could help a person to fall asleep. But there wasn't very much evidence. There were few controlled studies that we could evaluate. . . . When I say we found few controlled studies, I mean we found few studies where the criteria for effectiveness were objectively analyzed. We were aware also of the risks that attend the use of antihistamines. Antihistamines, introduced originally for the relief of allergic phenomena such as hay fever or allergic reactions to ingested foods or drugs, have side effects that cause drowsiness, and it is, of course, a side effect of the antihistamines that has been used for the treatment of sleeplessness. We were aware that antihistamines could make a person less able to operate machinery, do motor tasks that are required in our civilization such as driving a car or walking carefully across a busy city street, or operating a dangerous machine safely. Knowing this, we believed that antihistamines might serve as over-the-counter sleep aids if additional studies adducing evidence of efficacy without undue adverse effects could be carried out. Such studies were to be carried out in sleep laboratories where effects on sleeplessness and the quality of sleep could be monitored. To sum up, we put the antihistamines in category III on the basis that there was not enough evidence for effectiveness, and that such evidence might be forthcoming if higher doses were used and if objective, well-planned studies were carried out. We wanted to see if, when the drug was used in higher doses, and if it were effective, it were also safe. This is a conservative and proper attitude to take for drugs marketed over the counter. . . .

I would like to finish with a few general comments. I think that if a suspicion exists about the ineffectiveness or the lack of safety of a drug or of both, it should be withdrawn. If this cannot be done because of the regulations under which the Food and Drug Administration operates, I think it appropriate that we do not advertise the drug. If, because of the constraints under which the Food and Drug Administration and the Federal Trade Commission operate, it is impossible to stop the drug from being marketed *and* advertised, I think we should put constraints upon advertising the drug such that descriptive information be available and that claims as to safety or effectiveness not be made beyond those found by the panel which carefully reviewed it. I say these things because I am very much aware of "the law's delay", a phrase from *Hamlet*, written almost 400 years ago. Why should the consumer pay for the law's delay? . . .

Finally, I'd like to make a pitch for consideration of alternatives to drugs. One alternative is to consider the possibility that we may not need drugs for trivial symptoms. I know that, according to the law, people have the right to take drugs. I know that we are a drug-taking society, that we are encouraged to take drugs, not only by advertising aimed at the consumer but also by advertising aimed at the medical profession. I think drugs are useful where the benefit-to-risk ratio is favorable, where the game is worth the candle. But I think the use of drugs for the relief of transient, minor symptoms is unwise and should not be encouraged. People should be made aware of the fact that occasional nervousness or anxiety is a normal part of living and does no harm. I think people also should be aware of the fact that occasional sleeplessness is a normal response to extra pressures, and if it is not persistent, does no harm. If the symptom is persistent the person should be carefully evaluated with regard to the cause of the sleeplessness and appropriate recommendations made. Signs and symptoms are often useful clues to the diagnosis and progress of disease. There are drugs that can suppress most all of them.

Lester C. Mark, M.D., Professor of Anesthesiology,
College of Physicians and Surgeons, Columbia University,
622 West 168th Street, New York, New York 10032

Our deliberations concentrated on the use of antihistamines, singly or in combination, as nighttime sleep-aids and daytime sedatives. These drugs have long been used by physicians for their antiallergic properties. A frequently observed side effect, namely sedation, was transformed into the desired therapeutic benefit for O.T.C. use. Unfortunately, in their laudable zeal for safety, most manufacturers chose doses of these drugs which ranged from moderately effective to threshold (or barely effective) to ineffective. Some combinations included more than one antihistamine, each in even lower dosage, hoping thereby to reduce toxicity while adding up to therapeutic efficacy. . . . We ended up by placing the antihistamines diphenhydramine, methapyrilene (either as the fumarate or the hydrochloride) and pyrilamine in Category III ("available data insufficient for final classification at present") for reasons of both safety and efficacy, with an additional period of three years for testing to achieve an appropriate dose which would be both safe and effective. During this time, the drugs would remain on the market. Two other antihistamines, doxylamine and phenyltoloxamine, were placed in a new "Category III with a marketing hold" designated as "Category III (MH)", since they are not currently available as O.T.C. nighttime sleep-aids and further testing is required to demonstrate their safety and efficacy for this use. . . .

The only remaining combinations, temporarily allowable in Category III with three years for testing as either nighttime sleep-aids or daytime sedatives, are those containing analgesics, which have meanwhile been referred to the O.T.C. Internal Analgesics Panel for evaluation of their analgesic claims.

Dr. William Lijinsky, Director, Chemical Carcinogenesis
Program, Frederick Cancer Research Center, Frederick,
Maryland.

Possible danger of over-the-counter drugs:
All substances which are effective drugs are biologically

active compounds. Many of them might have, in addition to the desirable action, less desirable ones about which we know little, and some of which might be dangerous. In particular there can be long term effects which might not be discovered for some time. The calamity of thalidomide is an example. However, in the case of drugs available only on prescription there is some control of possible adverse effects because of the limited intake of these medicines.

Over-the-counter drugs, including cold remedies and sleeping aids, can be bought and taken in large quantities, even though the dose is carefully recommended. These compounds, therefore, represent a source of danger if they happen to have side effects which are not well known or are undiscovered. Most of the over-the-counter sleep aids and many of the cold remedies contain antihistaminics, all of which are secondary or tertiary amines. One of the most common is methapyrilene, but chlorpheniramine and others are frequently used, although at lower doses than methapyrilene. A usual composition of a sleep aid tablet is 25 milligrams of methapyrilene.

Methapyrilene, like many similar antihistaminic drugs, is a tertiary amine. Being a tertiary amine it reacts with nitrites in mildly acid solution to form a nitrosamine, dimethylnitrosamine, which is one of the most potent carcinogens known, inducing liver cancer in rats. There are other products of the reaction which have not been identified. The formation of dimethylnitrosamine takes place over a wide range of concentrations, and some dimethylnitrosamine can be identified even at quite low concentrations of methapyrilene and nitrite.

A favored site of reaction of methapyrilene with nitrite is in the stomach, where the mildly acid medium facilitates the formation of dimethylnitrosamine.

The formation of nitrosamines from methapyrilene and several similar drugs by reaction with nitrite in mildly acid solution has been demonstrated. The amount of dimethylnitrosamine formed from methapyrilene under these conditions decreases at lower concentrations, but will never become zero. In other words, some dimethylnitrosamine will be formed at all concentrations, provided that the medium is mildly acid.

Ernest Hartmann, M.D., Director, Sleep and Dream
Laboratory, Boston State Hospital, and Professor of
Psychiatry, Tufts University School of Medicine, 591 Morton
St., Boston, Massachusetts 02124

First of all, I believe that in a more ideal society, towards
which we may gradually strive, the present distinction between illegal drugs, drugs to be sold under prescription only,
and drugs available over-the-counter, (OTC) would be unnecessary. If adult citizens were sufficiently educated and
well-informed, and labeling was sufficiently accurate, it
might be quite possible to allow any medication to be sold
over-the-counter, and one could rely on the good sense of the
consumer to buy only what was necessary and safe. However,
in the present state of our society, such an ideal situation does
not exist, and I therefore agree that the consumer requires a
certain amount of protection. I agree that under present
circumstances only certain drugs should be available over-
the-counter, and the consumer has the right to expect that
these drugs have been carefully screened for safety and
efficacy and to make sure that the benefits outweigh the risks.

The panel made many specific recommendations which
I will not review in detail, but overall the suggestions of the
panel were usually that unnecessary and unsafe ingredients
be removed from the medication available. Thus if the
panel's recommendations are followed, OTC sleep aids and
sedatives would generally consist of a single ingredient—an
antihistamine; while OTC stimulants would consist of a
single stimulant substance—caffeine. I agree with these
recommendations, and with the medical principle behind
them—that wherever possible a single chemical substance or
ingredient should be used to treat a single condition or
complaint. The addition of further ingredients produces
hazards both in terms of specific problems of safety of the
additional ingredients, and in terms of multiple known and
unknown interactions between the drug constituents and
various other substances frequently present in the body,
including alcohol, nicotine, marijuana, foods, etc. that may be
taken simultaneously. Since it is unrealistic to predict and
study each possible interaction in detail, the general principle is that mixtures of substances not be used unless one can
clearly establish their superiority over a single ingredient in
an appropriate population. . . .

I would like to call the sub-committee's attention to an important statement in our report concerning labeling and advertising. The panel suggested certain principles for labeling of these over-the-counter products—specifically that the claims made should correspond simply and specifically to the results of particular studies which had demonstrated positive results. For instance, if it has been carefully established by sleep studies such as we have recommended, that a drug reduces time to sleep in insomniac adults, this should be stated on the label; but the label should not make vague claims about "improved sleep" or "more refreshing sleep" which cannot be adequately defined or tested. . . .

My laboratory and a number of others have been doing research concerning a food substance—the amino acid l-tryptophan—and have found that this naturally occuring food substance induces sleep effectively if taken in pure form. At this point further testing is still required, but I consider it quite possible that this substance will turn out to be an effective and unusually safe sleeping medication which should perhaps be sold over-the-counter in a few year's time. Thus, I believe a continuing mechanism to consider possible drugs, perhaps a mechanism somewhat similar to our panel, would be useful. . . .

The cost of performing complete safety and efficacy studies of a new drug is now usually several million dollars. I agree that extensive testing is usually necessary, but this cost alone already raises barriers for small companies. In addition, the restraint-of-trade laws are interpreted in such a way that several companies are not allowed to pool resources for the testing of a new drug. Nor, apparently, are companies permitted to divide the work so that each will have to bear only a portion of the cost of testing. This obviously leads to a situation where only a large company can be successful, and a situation where only definitely patentable substances or combinations will be developed. For instance, my laboratory has pursued studies of the natural amino acid l-tryptophan from a theoretical point of view. Recently, since we have shown that l-tryptophan can act as a sleeping medication, several pharmaceutical companies have shown some interest. However, in each case companies concluded that it would not be worth their while to spend huge sums developing a medication for which they would be unable to obtain exclusive patent rights. By chance, I have just heard that one company has recently obtained a patent on l-tryptophan combined with propranolol, an adrenergic blocker, as a potential sleeping pill. This combination strikes me as potentially quite dangerous; it seems to me obvious that propranolol was added since the combination would be patentable whereas l-tryptophan alone was not.

I am not a lawyer, and cannot make detailed suggestions, but I believe that some change in the laws governing restraint-of-trade and patents could be beneficial to the drug industry and to the health of the American public.

Evaluating The Most Popular
Prescription Sleeping Pills

Drug	Generic Name	Manufacturer	Type of Drug
Dalmane	Flurazepam hydrochloride	Roche	Hypnotic (sleeping pill). Related chemically to tranquilizers such as Librium and Valium.

Drug	Generic Name	Manufacturer	Type of Drug
Luminal, Stental (widely prescribed under generic name)	Phenobarbital Sodium	Winthrop (Luminal) Robins (Stental) and others	Sedative-hypnotic barbiturate

Action	Adverse Reaction	Precautions
On CNS; reduces responses to stimulation. Acts within 20 minutes. For all types of insomnia, induces sleep for seven to eight hours; no dependence reported, but may cause dependence after prolonged use.	Reported seven percent of users; includes dizziness, excessive drowsiness, staggering, loss of muscle coordination, falling (especially in the old and weak); lethargy, severe sedation, disorientation, coma (possibly due to overdose or drug intolerance) have been reported. Also: headache, heartburn, nausea, diarrhea, vomiting, constipation, chest, stomach, and/or joint pains, nervousness, talkativeness, apprehension, irritability, weakness, palpitations, pain in urinary tract. Rare: sweating, flushes, blurred vision, shortness of breath, skin rash, dry mouth, appetite loss, euphoria, depression, slurred speech, confusion, restlessness, hallucinations, paradoxical reactions such as excitement, stimulation, and hyperactivity.	Do not take alcohol or other CNS depressants because of additive effect; avoid any task requiring mental alertness shortly after taking the drug—do not drive, operate machinery. Not recommended for people under 15, pregnant women (safety of Dalmane not established).
Action	**Adverse Reaction**	**Precautions**
CNS depressant, long-acting sedative-hypnotic; widely used as daytime sedative; in hypnotic doses, sleep generally occurs in ½ to one hour and lasts six to 10 hours; because it counteracts spasm it is used in convulsive disorders.	Lassitude, rash, vertigo, hangover, nausea, diarrhea, excitement, fever, delirium, but these idiosyncratic reactions are not common.	May be habit-forming; see BUTISOL; administration of this drug should be carefully controlled by a physician; in patients with impaired kidney or liver functions, dosage should be reduced.

Drug	Generic Name	Manufacturer	Type of Drug
Butisol Sodium	Sodium Butabarbital	McNeil	Barbiturate sedative-hypnotic, used as much for daytime sedation as for nighttime sleep.
Drug	Generic Name	Manufacturer	Type of Drug
Noctec, Aquachloral Kessodrate (widely prescribed under generic name)	Chloral hydrate	Squibb (Noctec), Webcon (Aquachloral), McKesson (Kessodrate), and others who sell drug under its generic name.	Sedative-hypnotic, nonbarbiturate
Drug	Generic Name	Manufacturer	Type of Drug
Tuinal	Secobarbital sodium and amobarbital sodium	Lilly	Hypnotic, barbiturate mixture

Action	Adverse Reaction	Precautions
Effective within 30 minutes; action continues for five to six hours; acts as CNS depressant and, depending on dose, will produce effects ranging from mild sedation to deep sleep. Coma and death may result from overdose.	Slight hangover, lethargy, drowsiness, skin eruptions, headache, nausea and vomiting, dizziness; allergic reactions such as local swelling or dermatitis may occur; some people, especially the elderly or debilitated, may suffer marked excitement or depression.	May be habit-forming: habituation precedes abuse, with first psychological, then physical dependence; extent of barbiturate addiction is unknown, but may possibly exceed heroin addiction; withdrawal, if sudden, can lead to severe condition, resembling epilepsy, and if untreated can result in high fever, coma, death; all chronic users must withdraw gradually from barbiturates under medical supervision; barbiturates potentiate effects of alcohol, non-barbiturate hypnotics, other CNS depressants, but decrease potency of drugs such as anticoagulants (their effectiveness must be checked); overdosage (accidental or intentional) can cause profound shock, respiratory depression, loss of reflexes, coma, death; social hazards include lack of mental alertness (avoid driving, operating machinery), accidental use by children.

Action	Adverse Reaction	Precautions
Sedative-hypnotic; CNS depressant action usually begins within 30 minutes and sleep within an hour; effect continues for four to six hours.	With exception of stomach upset, few unfavorable side effects, according to Squibb; excitement and delirium are rarely encountered; tolerance and addiction are quite uncommon.	May be habit-forming; effect on blood-clotting must be evaluated when taking anticoagulants; should not be taken by people with severe liver, kidney, heart disease; alcohol potentiates sedative-hypnotic effects.

Action	Adverse Reaction	Precautions
CNS depressant, is moderately long-acting hypnotic; not recommended for continuous daytime sedation.	Paradoxical reaction in the form of excitement, hangover, pain, may appear; hypersensitivity reactions.	May be habit forming; must be used with caution by people with liver disease, since this might prolong the hypnotic effect.

Drug	Generic Name	Manufacturer	Type of Drug
Quaalude	Methaqualone	Rorer	Nonbarbiturate sedative-hypnotic

Drug	Generic Name	Manufacturer	Type of Drug
Doriden	Glutethimide	USV Pharma-ceutical	Nonbarbiturate hypnotic

Action	Adverse Reaction	Precautions
Mechanism and CNS area of action unknown; does not work like barbiturates; drowsiness occurs within 10 to 20 minutes.	Headache, hangover, fatigue, dizziness, transient paresthesia (peculiar sensations) in extremities; occasionally, restlessness, anxiety; dry mouth, lack of appetite, vomiting, stomach discomfort, diarrhea; various allergic skin problems; rarely, serious anemia.	May be habit-forming; manufacturer reports occasional psychological dependence, rarely physical dependence (addiction); because of rapid action, should be taken only at bedtime, immediately before retiring; not recommended for children; decreased mental alertness precludes driving, operating dangerous machinery. Avoid other sedatives, painkillers, psychiatric drugs, alcohol, because of possible additive effects; should not be used for longer than three months; should be avoided by addiction-prone people, those who increase dosage on their own initiative.
Action	Adverse Reaction	Precautions
Hypnotic, CNS depressant. Induces sleep usually within 30 minutes; duration of action generally four to eight hours. Recommended by manufacturer for those with difficulty falling asleep and those who awaken too often during the night.	Generalized skin rash suggests drug must be stopped; other types of skin eruptions; rarely, nausea, hangover, blurring of vision; paradoxical excitement, serious blood disorders.	May be habit-forming: withdrawal symptoms include nausea, abdominal discomfort, convulsions, delirium; newborn infants of mothers dependent on Doriden may exhibit withdrawal symptoms; to be prescribed to pregnant women only if potential benefits exceed possible hazards; not recommended for children under 12; do not take with alcohol or other CNS depressants because of additive effect; watch concomitant use of anticoagulant drugs; avoid tasks requiring mental alertness shortly after taking drug—do not drive, operate machinery; avoid less than four hours before arising.

Drug	Generic Name	Manufacturer	Type of Drug
Placidyl	Ethchlorvynol	Abbott	Hypnotic, nonbarbiturate

Drug	Generic Name	Manufacturer	Type of Drug
Nembutal	Pentobarbital sodium	Abbott	Barbiturate sedative-hypnotic

Drug	Generic Name	Manufacturer	Type of Drug
Seconal	Secobarbital sodium	Lilly	Sedative-hypnotic barbiturate

Action	Adverse Reaction	Precautions
Considered short-acting hypnotic; acts on CNS, inducing sleep within 15 minutes to one hour. Effective for approximately five hours. More useful for the insomniac who has trouble falling asleep than the one who has trouble staying asleep.	Mild hangover, mild excitation; low blood pressure, nausea and vomiting, upset stomach, aftertaste, blurring of vision, dizziness, facial numbness, allergic reactions; rarely, jaundice, blood disorder.	May be habit-forming; do not take with alcohol, barbiturates, tranquilizers, or other CNS depressants; avoid tasks requiring mental alertness—do not drive or operate machinery.

Action	Adverse Reaction	Precautions
A short-to-intermediate-acting barbiturate, exerts its effects within 15 to 30 minutes, with effects lasting from three to six hours; acts as CNS depressant.	Mild to severe breathing problems, circulatory collapse, skin rash and other allergic reactions; lethargy, residual sedation (hangover effect); nausea, vomiting; paradoxial excitement.	May be habit-forming; as dependence develops, people tend to increase dosage; abrupt stopping of drug causes withdrawal symptoms; chronic user must withdraw gradually; like other barbiturates, potentiates effect of alcohol, decreases effectiveness of drugs such as anticoagulants.

Action	Adverse Reaction	Precautions
Central nervous system depressant, short-acting sedative-hypnotic; depending on dose, will produce response ranging from mild sedation to deep sleep; used more often for insomnia than daytime sedation.	Paradoxical excitement, hangover, or pain; varied allergic reactions occur on occasion.	See Luminal

A Summary Description of Common Sleep Disorders

Courtesy of Sleep-Wake Disorders Unit,
Montefiore Hospital and Medical Center, New York, N.Y.

Sleep Apneas

Sleep apnea is a condition in which the patient has frequent cessations of breathing during sleep. These cessations may last from 20 to 130 seconds. Apneas are classified as central, upper airway obstructive, or mixed, to aid diagnosis. Central apnea is a transient halt in the regular movement of the diaphragm. Upper airway obstructive apnea is the development of a functional obstruction through collapse of tissue structures of the upper airway which prevents breathing, although the diaphragm contracts to take a breath. Mixed apnea is a central followed by an upper airway obstructive apnea. Sleep apnea patients characteristically have heavy snoring as a symptom.

Sleep apnea may cause several hundred brief or sometimes prolonged arousals during a night. This may produce a significant insomnia. The patient does not realize that he has these apneic episodes but may complain of insomnia or a disturbed sleep. Apnea may also cause sleepers to spend all their sleep in light Stage I or II of NREM sleep so that they do not get enough Stage III and IV sleep. Such apneic sufferers complain of excessive daytime sleepiness and sleep attacks and are diagnosed as hypersomniacs with sleep apnea.

Apneic hypersomnia is sometimes correlated with obesity, and when severe, this may develop into the Pickwickian syndrome. Pickwickian syndrome is a condition in which the patient suffers upper airway obstructive sleep apnea, leading to chronic insufficient breathing (hypoventilation), low blood oxygen content (hypoxia), excessive daytime sleepiness and sleep attacks, pulmonary hypertension, disease of the right side of the heart (cor pulmonale), and possible systemic hypertension and right heart failure.

Ondine's Curse is a form of sleep apnea in which the

patient's breathing may stop completely during sleep. If cessation of breathing does not wake the sleeper, he may die. This condition is usually caused by a tumor or lesion in the brainstem or upper spinal cord. (Ondine was a water nymph of German legend, who laid a curse on a lover who spurned her that he should "forget" to breathe when not consiously willing it.) Ondine's Curse must be treated by mechanically assisted breathing during sleep.

It is conservatively estimated that sleep apnea may afflict at least 50,000 persons in the U.S. Because chronic sleep apnea often produces hypertension, researchers have postulated that the estimate might run much higher if all hypertensive patients were screened for sleep apnea. The increasing number of persons appearing in sleep disorders centers with sleep apnea also suggests that the actual incidence might be much higher than previous estimates.

One study has estimated that one to five percent of insomniacs suffer from sleep apnea. This apnea tends to be of the central type. Fifteen to 20 percent of hypersomnia patients seen in the study had sleep apnea, usually of the mixed or upper airway obstructive classes. About 85 percent of sleep apnea patients are male. Symptoms usually appear after age 40.

Apnea is common in the premature and full-term infant and has been theorized to be universal in infants one to three months old. It is even more commonly seen in premature infants and seems related to birth weight. Apnea has been related to sudden infant death syndrome (SIDS), to be described later. Older children with apneas often also have enuresis (bedwetting).

To diagnose apnea, physicians may question the patient's bed partner to find out if the patient snores especially heavily and with snorting. The loud, heavy, snorting snore is the resumption of breathing after an apnea.

The physician may also ask the patient to go to sleep in his office for an hour or so, wearing a respiratory gauge. Breathing stoppages of central apnea will show up on the gauge. Many central apnea sufferers may sleep several hours without apnea attacks, however, and apnea may be absent on any one day. Therefore the diagnosis of apnea is best confirmed by referral to a sleep disorders center.

Apnea is easily detected in a sleep disorders clinic, because the patient may have 400-500 episodes per night. The respiration measurement used in such clinics detects cessation of diaphragm movements. Air flow meters over the nostrils and mouth distinguish upper airway obstructive apnea by showing no air movement in the presence of strong efforts to breathe, as indicated by the chest respiration gauge. The oximeter on the ear lobe detects a falloff in the oxygen content of the blood as a result of an apnea. The respiratory control centers in the brain interrupt a central or obstructive apnea before hypoxia (lack of oxygen) becomes severe. However, the upper airway obstructive type resists efforts by the diaphragm to restore breathing for longer periods, and the hypoxia is much more severe. Such apneas have been recorded to last for two to 2½ minutes.

Hypersomniac apnea patients complain about excessive daytime sleepiness. This may result from lack of restful sleep, because of the frequent transient arousals. In addition, it is possible that the buildup of carbon dioxide in the blood during the recurring nighttime upper airway obstructive apnea may blunt the chemoreceptors that stimulate respiration. Thus hypoventilation may persist into the day, because chemoreceptors send inadequate signals for involuntary breathing to respiratory centers in the brain. A vicious cycle may thus be set up: hypoventilation during the day continues the hypoxic state with persistent high levels of carbon dioxide in the blood, especially during sleep at night.

Hypersomniac apnea patients often have many short sleep periods lasting only a few seconds during the day—microsleeps. They find themselves able to perform simple routine, repetitive tasks, although sleepy, but not complex acts during hypersomniac episodes with microsleeps. Frequent microsleeps during the day may cause periods of apparent amnesia and inappropriate behavior, in which the patient cannot recall his activities during certain periods.

Hypersomniac apnea patients are difficult to rouse fully from a night's sleep, even by painful stimuli. When they do awaken, they seem disoriented as to place and time and have problems with visual perception. These periods of "foggy mind" may last 15 minutes to an hour.

Eventually, hypersomniac obstructive sleep apnea can

lead to pulmonary hypertension, heart disease of the right side of the heart (cor pulmonale), right heart failure, cardiac arrthythmias, and systemic hypertension. In one study, 60 percent of adults and 62 percent of children with hypersomniac apnea were found to have hypertension. In the Pickwickian syndrome, characterized by obesity in addition to hypersomniac apnea, these complications are especially frequent.

Hypersomniac symptoms have led children and teenagers in rare instances to be wrongly classed as mentally retarded. On the other hand, continuous hypoxia of hypersomniac apnea persisting undiagnosed from infancy has been reported to cause actual mental retardation.

As with insomniac apnea, the physician may try to detect apnea and characteristic snoring in his office and question the patient's bed partner about snoring. However, definitive diagnosis should be made in a sleep disorders center, where procedures can also be performed to diagnose the complications of this syndrome. Such special techniques include the insertion of a catheter from a vein in the forearm, through the heart, and into the pulmonary artery to detect pulmonary hypertension.

Insomniac apnea, characterized by central apnea, has been treated with some success with chlorimipramine. This drug is currently available in the U.S. for investigational use only. Hypnotic (sleep inducing) drugs should not be prescribed for apneic insomniacs, because the apnea results from a defect in the mechanism that stimulates respiration, and this mechanism can be depressed further by hypnotics, making the problem worse.

Hypersomniac apnea, where upper airway obstruction is crucial, can sometimes be alleviated in children by surgical removal of tonsils and adenoids. An intrathoracic goiter, growing within the chest rather than outward, has on rare occasions been found to aggravate upper airway apnea, and its removal has benefited the patient.

If surgery does not help, and if the apnea is severe enough to cause the complications described above, the sleep disorders clinic may perform or recommend a tracheostomy. A tracheostomy is an opening made into the patient's trachea (windpipe) through the skin to bypass upper airway structures that collapse and obstruct during sleep. The patient can close the tracheostomy opening during the day and therefore speak normally, and open it only at night for sleep. Following tracheostomy, hypersomnia disappears in one or two days. The irregular heart rhythms and hypertension also subside after two to three months. In a year of follow up, the frequency of nighttime central apnea in these patients is also normally reduced in frequency. This last finding lends support to the idea that hypoxia of upper airway apnea contributes to a vicious cycle of increased frequency of apnea which may be due to blunting of chemoreceptors.

Chlorimipramine has also been used with some success with hypersomniac apnea.

Pickwickian syndrome can be treated in part by major weight loss. After weight loss, central apneas may still occur, but with less frequency. Symptoms of hypersomnia also decrease in intensity. Alternatively, oral progesterone or medroxyprogesterone acetate have also been tried but their efficacy requires further careful evaluation.

Future research may add powerful, new diagnostic procedures for sleep apneas to the sleep disorders clinician's armamentarium. These advances are expected to come from better correlation of apneic incidents with specific states of sleep, REM and NREM, and a better understanding of the mechanism of the apnea episode. This improved correlation could lead to a reclassification of the sleep apneas on a more logical basis than the observation of an external clinical sign, such as obesity in Pickwickian syndrome.

Sudden Infant Death Syndrome (SIDS)

SIDS is the death of an infant in its crib with no signs of suffocation, distress, or other cause. One major theory is that it is caused by a fatal apnea during sleep. SIDS causes 10,000 infant deaths yearly in the United States and is the leading cause of death in the first six months of life. Most victims are two to four months old, premature or of lower-than-normal birth weight, and come from low socioeconomic levels of society. They often have a respiratory infection at the time of death. Most deaths occur at night during the sleep period and in winter months.

Infants have been resuscitated after what were thought to be "near misses." In the hospital they are then monitored for breathing to detect a recurrence and may be found to have apnea. Survivors usually grow up normally without further difficulty—but further study is needed to determine whether these may develop adult sleep apnea syndrome.

Siblings of SIDS victims have been found to be five times as likely as the normal population of infants to suffer SIDS also. Physicians theorize that certain environmental factors and events of normal development may combine to exacerbate an inherited tendency to abnormal, sleep-related respiratory drive.

Narcolepsy

Narcolepsy is a sleep disorder mainly characterized by frequent, almost uncontrollable attacks of daytime sleep. In contrast to the excessive daytime sleepiness of the hypersomnias to be described later, narcoleptic impulses to sleep are almost irresistable. Classical narcolepsy consists of four symptoms. The first is the occurrence of as many as 15-20 sleep attacks daily, each usually lasting less than 15 minutes. The second is cataplexy, which is a daytime attack of muscle weakness involving collapse of the body resulting from loss of muscle tone, often triggered by emotional situations. In cataplexy, the eyes may sometimes remain open and the person is always aware of his surroundings during the several seconds to one-to-two-minutes that the attack lasts. The third symptom is auditory and/or visual hallucinations called hypnagogic hallucinations, so called because they occur at the onset of, or on waking from, nighttime sleep. The fourth is sleep paralysis which occurs at the onset of, or on waking from nighttime sleep, in which the patient is unable to move his body muscles.

A recent survey of 3,000 physicians revealed that 0.6 percent of patients seen have narcolepsy, with the incidence in family practice and internal medicine reaching 0.9-1.0 percent. It is estimated that only about one-third of the several hundred thousand narcoleptics in the U.S. have been diagnosed, and that the mean time from onset of a symptom to diagnosis is 15 years. Tendency to narcolepsy is apparently inherited, because close relatives of narcoleptics are 20 times more likely than the general population to develop symptoms.

Of several hundred narcoleptics in one study, all suffered daytime sleep attacks, while 70 percent also had cataplectic attacks. Twenty-five percent experienced hypnagogic hallucinations and 50 percent suffered sleep paralysis. Only ten percent had all four symptoms. Laughter triggered 94 percent of the cataplectic attacks; anger, 86 percent; amusement, 70 percent; athletic activity, 60 percent; excitement, 56 percent; elation, 52 percent; attempts to resist sleep attacks, 50 percent; surprise, 48 percent; tension, 44 percent; a call to action, 34 percent; and sexual activity, 32 percent.

Symptoms of narcolepsy often appear at puberty, usually as daytime sleep attacks. It has been suggested that the problem may be related to hormonal changes occurring during this developmental phase. Cataplexy may not appear for four to five years after sleep attacks begin, and in rare instances not until 30 years after. Once established, the symptoms are lifelong and often disabling.

Relatives, employers, and narcoleptics themselves have often concluded that the sufferer is merely "lazy," thus delaying a proper diagnosis. This stigma may account for the incidence of depression in 29 percent of one sample of narcoleptics with sleep attacks and of 17 percent in those with cataplexy as well. However, the disorder itself may also produce a certain tendency to depression. Physicians diagnosing narcolepsy should often test for hypothyroidism, hypoglycemia, emotional problems, or other sleep disorders to be described later, such as Kleine-Levin and apneic hypersomnia syndrome.

In the sleep laboratory, the most common diagnostic feature of narcolepsy is the presence of REM sleep at the onset of a nighttime sleep period. In normal persons, sleep begins with a NREM period, and REM appears only after about 90 minutes. Narcolepsy has been explained in terms of an intrusion of REM sleep phenomena into the waking state. Thus daytime sleep attacks are usually attacks of REM sleep. Cataplexy and sleep paralysis may result from an inappropriate triggering of skeletal muscle tone inhibition that normally occurs in REM sleep. Hypnagogic hallucinations may also be caused by dreamlike REM mental activity occurring inappropriately in the waking state.

Preliminary findings from one center in a small number of patients indicate that there may be four types of narcolepsy, characterized by disorder of the REM mechanism only, disorder of the NREM mechanism only, major REM disorder and minor NREM disorder, and major NREM and minor REM disorder.

Once diagnosed, narcoleptics, their families, and their employers should be counselled by physicians about the nature of the disease and its control by medication. Stimulants such as methylphenidate, pemoline, and dextroamphetamine, drugs that are known to suppress REM sleep in normal persons, can be prescribed to prevent sleep attacks. Drugs such as imipramine or protriptyline may prevent cataplexy. The anticataplectic effect of these drugs seem unrelated to their antidepressant activity, however. In addition, psychotherapy may be necessary to treat the effects on patients' personalities of years of living with their misunderstood condition. Doses of drugs should be gauged carefully to avoid psychiatric or neurological side effects. Some physicians have urged caution in prescribing the stimulants together with the antidepressants, because theoretically they could interact to cause hypertension. Other physicians point out, however, that these two drug classes are routinely used together to manage narcolepsy without incident. One therapeutic regimen advises use of stimulants only periodically when the patient expects situations that may trigger sleep attacks. Tricyclic antidepressant drugs may produce sexual impotence as a side effect in men. Clinicians are divided as to whether to advise withdrawal of these drugs at intervals to allow normal sexual activity.

Isolated Sleep Paralysis

Sleep paralysis is one of the classic symptoms of narcolepsy, but this symptom also occurs alone in rare cases, and may be a separate sleep disorder. As in sleep paralysis of narcolepsy, the sufferer is able to move only his eyes and breathe.

Isolated sleep paralysis is common among Canadian Eskimos, who explain it as attempts of possession by spirits. Among these people, it may be an inherited tendency or a hysterical symptom, caused by the repression of anger required by Eskimo culture. Further research may determine whether the sleep paralysis present in such high incidence in Eskimos is identical with the REM sleep mechanism defect known to Western Medicine. If so, studies among Eskimos may shed further light on the inheritance and management of this disorder.

Drug therapy does not seem to be indicated for isolated sleep paralysis. Affected persons can will the termination of such attacks by vigorous movement of their eyeballs, attempts to blink the eyelids, followed by moving facial muscles, progressing to more distant muscles. Counselling by physicians may help patients to understand their condition and the means of ending the attack.

Painful Nocturnal Erection Syndrome

Penile erections normally occur in 80-90 percent of REM sleep periods. In some persons, nocturnal erection is painful, often waking the sleeper. Erection in the waking state is not painful for these persons, however. Painful nocturnal erection syndrome may or may not be a disorder of the REM sleep mechanism. There is no treatment known for the condition. The cause is unknown. Physicians should counsel patients, reassuring them that the syndrome has no effect on normal sexual activity.

Night Terror Attacks

Night terror (pavor nocturnus) is characterized by the sleeper suddenly sitting up in bed, awakening from sleep, screaming and moaning, eyes open, pale, and with a terrified expression. Episodes can last 15-30 minutes, during which the sufferer moans and cries out frightening, bizarre phrases. Following an attack, the patient usually goes right back to sleep and does not remember the episode in the morning.

A night terror attack is not identical with a nightmare. Night terrors characteristically occur during Stage III or IV sleep, the deepest stages of NREM sleep, whereas nightmares, which are "bad dreams," occur during REM and can be remembered afterward. Night terror may be associated with sleepwalking, sleep talking, and bedwetting in children, and like these other sleep disorders is thought to be related to the child's immature nervous system.

Night terrors usually begin at age four to five and end about age seven or eight. A survey of 3,000 physicians revealed that night terrors occurred in 1.2 percent of all patients seen. Among physicians of various individual specialties, incidences were family practitioners, general practitioners, and internists, 1.5-1.8 percent; pediatricians, 4.0 percent; and psychiatrists and child psychiatrists, 3.7-4.9 percent.

Physicians should counsel parents that their children will probably outgrow this condition, that it is not caused by daytime worry or stress, and that it does not produce any carryover into waking life. Night terrors in adults also known as "incubus" may be caused by emotional problems, and a psychiatric evaluation is indicated. Diazepam is often successful in reducing the incidence of night terror. This drug is known to suppress Stage III and IV sleep. Because the effect of chronic use of psychoactive drugs or the suppression of any sleep state in children is unknown, physicians do not recommend the chronic use of diazepam for children. Night terror sometimes occurs as a symptom in epilepsy, and in such cases appropriate anticonvulsant medication has been used successfully.

Somnambulism (Sleepwalking)

Sleep walking is associated with sleep talking, bedwetting, and night terror, usually in children. Like these other sleep disorders, it may be due to immaturity of the child's nervous system. Sleep researchers believe that most children have a tendency to sleepwalk, and estimate that 15 percent of all children have walked at least once. It is apparently an inherited tendency, and most chronic sleepwalkers are male.

In a survey of 3,000 physicians, sleepwalkers comprised 0.6 percent of patients seen. Among physicians of various specialties, incidences were internists, family and general practitioners, 1.0-1.3 percent; and pediatricians, psychiatrists, and child psychiatrists, 2.0-2.3 percent.

Children usually outgrow sleepwalking. In adults, frequent sleepwalking is usually associated with emotional problems. In one study, 35 percent of chronic adult sleepwalkers were overtly schizophrenic, 28 percent were schizoid, and several individuals were neurotic.

The sleepwalker's eyes may be open but glassy and unseeing. The walker can navigate about a house, but lacks critical judgment. Thus he or she may fall over furniture, downstairs, or even through windows. Sleepwalking usually takes place in the first one-third of a night when sleep Stages III and IV predominate. EEG recordings done while the patient is sleepwalking show alpha waves, usually characteristic of relaxed waking, combined with low-frequency waves typical of Stages III and IV sleep. A sleep walk may be an actual walk for five to 30 minutes, or a mere sitting up in bed for 15-30 seconds. Because dreams occur during REM sleep and sleepwalking in NREM, the sleepwalker is *not* acting out a dream.

Physicians should counsel parents of sleepwalking children that they will probably outgrow the condition, that it does not indicate emotional problems, and that it will not have emotional effects on children's later lives. Parents should take steps to protect such children by locking windows and room doors and blocking stairways. While some persons have tied themselves by ropes to their beds, sleepwalkers often acquire the skill to untie the ropes without waking. Diazepam and imipramine have been successful in reducing sleepwalking, though their chronic use in children is not recommended. Physicians should rule out epilepsy when diagnosing sleepwalking. Psychiatric evaluation is indicated for chronic sleepwalking in adults.

Behavioral modification has been reported successful in controlling sleepwalking. Hypnotic suggestion reduced sleepwalking in four of six soldiers. One wife stopped her husband from sleepwalking by whistling derisively every time he rose from bed. Deep muscle relaxation training through EMG biofeedback has reduced high sleeping muscle tension in some sleepwalkers and reduced the frequency of sleepwalking.

Somniloquy (Sleep Talking)

Sleep talking is more common in children than adults. The talk is usually incomprehensible. Frequent, purposeful, understandable sleep talking and somnambulism in adults indicates emotional problems. Physicians should counsel parents that somniloquy does not indicate psychiatric problems in their children, and that they will probably outgrow it. Somniloquy may also be an inherited tendency. Diazepam has reduced frequency of somniloquy, but psychoactive drugs are not recommended for chronic use in children.

Enuresis (Bedwetting)

Enuresis can be primary or secondary. Primary enuresis is persistent bedwetting beyond what seems to be a normal age in children—four to five years. Secondary enuresis is a return of bedwetting after months or years in children who have learned continence. Primary enuresis is presumed to be caused by late maturation of the nervous system or of adequate bladder capacity and control. Primary enuresis can have organic causes, however, such as urethral obstruction in males, ectopic (displaced) ureter in females, diverticulum (presence of a pouch in) the anterior urethra, epispadias (opening of the urethra into a groove on the upper side of the penis or a fissure in the upper wall of the female urethra), ectopia vesicae (bladder malformation), or infection with cystitis. Secondary enuresis is usually indicative of emotional problems, but can be caused by diabetes or a neurological disease.

Children usually outgrow bedwetting at four years, though enuresis persists in 10-15 percent at four to five years; 10 percent at seven; three percent at 12; and one to three percent at 17-28 years (U.S. and British army studies). Among 3,000 physicians answering one survey, incidence of enuresis was 1.8 percent of all patients seen. Among specialties, incidence in patients of internists, family and general practitioners was 1.3-2.4 percent; of pediatricians and child psychiatrists, 9.6-10.7 percent; and of psychiatrists, 3.6 percent. It is the most common childhood sleep disorder and affects mostly boys.

The urination episode occurs in the first part of the night, usually with the end of a period of Stage III or IV of NREM sleep and a shift to Stage I or II. Because dreaming occurs in REM sleep, the bedwetter is not acting out a dream. If the person wets the bed, then passes into REM sleep, however, wetness may be incorporated into a dream. This coincidence has led to the erroneous association of bedwetting and dream content.

Physicians should counsel parents to handle enuresis tactfully so that no emotional burden is added to the child's late outgrowing of it. For children 10-12 years old going to camp or on a visit, imipramine, which reduces enuresis, may be prescribed. Chronic prescribing of imipramine in children is not advised by physicians, however. The drug seems to act by reducing stimulation of the bladder rather than by its antidepressant effect.

Parents may practice behavioral modification for children through use of a blanket that triggers a bell or buzzer when the child wets. Such a measure should be used with care and compassion, however, and only under guidance from a behavioral therapist thoroughly experienced in the technique. Immature, inadequate bladder capacity may be increased by urging the child to hold his urine as long as is bearable during the day, reinforcing the behavioral effect by keeping a chart of the increasing amount of urine the child can hold before pressure becomes unbearable.

Bruxism (Tooth Grinding)

Bruxism is a daytime habit and/or sleep disorder that can result in wear on teeth. Tooth loss and damage to the gums can eventually result. Bruxism occurs in Stage I or II NREM sleep, preceded by such symptoms of arousal as K-complexes in the EEG, increased heart rate, and vasoconstriction. Daytime bruxism can be "unlearned" through EMG biofeedback-guided behavior modification. Bruxism of sleep is usually treated by the wearing of rubber tooth guards. A U.S. Army study reported successful treatment of bruxism during sleep in 75 percent of 33 soldiers by EMG-guided biofeedback, but relapse rates are not known, and clinicians have doubts about the effectiveness of this daytime training on bruxism of sleep.

Jactatio Capitis Nocturna

Jactatio capitis nocturna is a violent, rhythmic hitting of the head against the pillow or rocking of the body as a ritual of going to sleep. It occurs in some infants and very young children. While classed as sleep disorder, the syndrome seems to cause no ill effects, does not appear to be symptomatic of a more fundamental neurological disorder, is eventually outgrown, and may be in the same class as thumb-sucking as a comforting habit. Persistence of this behavior into adulthood indicates the need for a neurological examination.

Nocturnal Myoclonus and Restless Legs Syndrome

Nocturnal myoclonus is a jerking or movement of the legs in a highly periodic manner every 25-40 seconds during sleep. Myoclonus has been estimated in one study to be the cause of 10-20 percent of chronic insomnia. Attacks may last for from minutes to several hours during sleep. The jerking motion often arouses the sleeper for about five to 15 seconds.

In severe cases there may be 300-400 such arousals during the night. In addition, the sleeping partner may move to a separate bed to avoid being kicked by the sleeper. Some sleep clinicians have theorized that nocturnal myoclonus may be caused by improper regulation of the REM sleep mechanism that suppresses skeletal muscle tone. According to this view, the jerks may be an overreaction to the inhibition.

Restless legs syndrome is the inability of the sleeper to keep his legs still while awake, but lying quietly in bed. This inability to lie still is also present during the day, but becomes noticeable when the patient tries to compose himself for sleep. Patients have reported uncomfortable, but not painful, creeping sensations deep in the muscles of the lower legs. These sensations sometimes also occur in the thighs and feet. The sufferer must often rise from bed to "walk off his legs" for 10-20 minutes. The resulting delay in finally getting to sleep results in complaints of sleep-onset insomnia. Patients with restless legs syndrome almost always have nocturnal myoclonus as well, though many persons with nocturnal myoclonus do not have the restless legs syndrome.

Patients are usually unaware of the jerking movements of nocturnal myoclonus. Physicians may suspect this disorder when the patient or his sleeping partner relates stories of the partner being kicked. In the sleep laboratory, attacks of myoclonus appear as an aroused EEG pattern. This lightened sleep, in addition to the frequent wakings, may contribute to the deteriorated quality of sleep. EMG recordings from the anterior tibialis muscle of the lower legs confirm the diagnosis of nocturnal myoclonus in all-night sleep recordings. Physicians may suspect restless legs syndrome from the patient's reports of insomnia and the creeping sensations of discomfort.

Diazepam has been prescribed to treat nocturnal myoclonus and restless legs syndrome with limited success. This drug may decrease the creeping sensations that compel the patient to get up and walk around. Diazepam is only partly effective against nocturnal myoclonus. In certain severe cases, it has been shown to reduce the number of wakings to 20-40 and also reduce the intensity of the jerks. Carbamazepine has also been used with some success with restless legs syndrome.

Hypersomnias

The hypersomnias are a constellation of sleep disorders involving excessive daytime sleepiness that are not caused by narcolepsy or sleep apnea syndrome. They are currently classified as the Kleine-Levin, neutral state, and subwakefulness syndrome, mixed hypersomnia, and idiopathic hypersomnia. In a recent study of 3,000 physicians, hypersomnias in general were found to comprise 3.2 percent of all patients seen. Among patients of individual specialties, incidences were internal medicine, family and general practice, 2.8-3.4 percent; psychiatry, 6.2 percent; and obstetrics and gynecology, 4.7 percent. Some forms of hypersomnia seem to be aggravated by pregnancy.

1. Kleine-Levin Syndrome

The Kleine-Levin syndrome is characterized by periods of severe hypersomnia, excessive eating, and excessive sex drive. Although it currently receives much attention from interested researchers in the medical literature, it is a very rare condition. Because androgens (male sex hormones) cause a similar condition, some sleep clinicians have theorized that it is caused by a hyperreactivity to androgens by the hypothalamus region of the brain, which may not have completely matured at puberty. Male patients tend to be young, schizoid, abnormally shy, and withdrawn. Female patients can experience the same or a similar condition before the onset of an irregular menstrual period.

Sleep laboratory studies have shown that sufferers get less Stage III and IV NREM sleep and less REM sleep than normal persons when the attack is present. In addition, REM periods may appear at the beginning of sleep, whereas in normal sleep, REM periods do not occur until about 90 minutes after sleep begins.

Lithium carbonate has been successful in preventing attacks in some patients but not in ending them. Symptoms in females disappear with the next regular period or after taking an estrogen/progesterone (female sex hormone) supplement.

2. Subwakefulness Syndrome

The subwakefulness syndrome is characterized by normal amounts of undisturbed nighttime sleep with normal amounts of deeper Stage III and IV NREM sleep and REM sleep, but hypersomnia all during the day. Patients have frequent periods of microsleeps during the day, lasting less than a minute. They thus have apparent lapses of memory and difficulty in concentration. Their cerebrospinal fluid contains abnormally low concentrations of homovanillic acid (HVA), a metabolic breakdown product of the neurotransmitter dopamine, when they are tested by administering the drug probenecid, which retards HVA elimination from cerebrospinal fluid.

This rare disorder is apparently a defect of the arousal mechanism of the brain. Investigations are underway to treat subwakefulness syndrome with dihydroxyphenylalanine (DOPA). DOPA is a compound which is converted to dopamine in the brain. Dopamine itself cannot cross the blood-brain barrier.

3. Neutral State Syndrome

Neutral state syndrome is another reported form of hypersomnia in which both sleep inducing and wakefulness mechanisms are disordered. Like patients with subwakefulness syndrome, those with neutral state syndrome suffer from excessive daytime sleepiness and fall into frequent microsleeps less than 60 seconds long. They can perform repetitive, routine tasks during hypersomniac periods, but not complex acts. They may later have amnesia about their activities at certain times of the day. Unlike patients with subwakefulness syndrome, persons with neutral state syndrome have aroused nighttime sleep with hundreds of microwakes lasting 10-60 seconds. Thus these patients are unable to maintain either the waking or sleeping state during the 24-hour period.

4. Mixed Hypersomnia

Mixed hypersomnia and narcolepsy may form a spectrum of related disorders according to certain sleep disorder specialists. Patients with mixed hypersomnia complain of excessive daytime sleepiness and may have cataplectic attacks. Evaluation in 24-hour sleep studies shows that daytime sleep periods sometimes begin with NREM and sometimes with REM. REM sleep onset is almost always seen in classical narcolepsy with cataplexy, whereas normal sleep begins with NREM. Whereas narcoleptics have disturbed, fragmented nighttime sleep, mixed hypersomniacs have an adequate amount of undisturbed sleep. When narcoleptics are deprived of sleep for a night, they have increased amounts of REM the next night. Mixed hypersomniacs have not been reported to show this REM rebound after sleep deprivation.

Thus both REM and NREM sleep mechanisms may be disturbed in mixed hypersomnia. As discussed before, there may be two types of mixed hypersomnia, classified according to which sleep mechanism is more disturbed, REM or NREM.

Mixed hypersomnia is usually treated with stimulants such as methylphenidate.

5. Idiopathic Narcolepsy

Idiopathic narcolepsy may be an additional component of the spectrum of sleep disorders that also includes classical narcolepsy-cataplexy and mixed hypersomnias. Idiopathic narcolepsy is characterized by daytime attacks of NREM sleep, according to certain specialists. Classical narcolepsy is characterized by REM sleep attacks. Mixed hypersomnias involve both REM and NREM daytime sleep attacks. Classical narcoleptic and mixed hypersomniac patients may have other narcoleptic symptoms, such as sleep paralysis, cataplexy, and hypnagogic hallucinations. Persons with idiopathic narcolepsy do not have these additional symptoms. Like other forms of narcolepsy and hypersomnia, idiopathic narcolepsy is also treated with stimulant drugs.

6. High 5-HIAA Hypersomnia

Some hypersomnia patients are found to have abnormally high levels of 5-hydroxyindoleacetic acid (5-HIAA) in their cerebrospinal fluid. 5-HIAA is a metabolic precursor of the neurotransmitter substance serotonin. Its presence in cerebrospinal fluid in abnormally high amounts may indicate higher amounts of serotonin than normal in the brain. Such patients have been successfully treated with inhibitors of serotonin such as methysergide.

7. Idiopathic Hypersomnia

Idiopathic hypersomnia is a diagnosis made when all other possible causes of hypersomnia have been ruled out. Patients with idiopathic hypersomnia complain of excessive length of nighttime sleep, which may last as long as 20 hours. Unlike those of narcolepsy, daytime sleep attacks of idiopathic hypersomnia are more easily resisted.

Other causes of hypersomnia which first must be ruled out are brain tumors, central nervous system defects, head injury, cerebrovascular disorder (such as stroke), emotional problems, or disturbance of normal biological rhythms. Idiopathic hypersomnia may occur as two types. In 33 percent of patients in one study, "sleep drunkenness" occurred on waking, lasting for 15 to 60 minutes. Sleep drunkenness is a mental confusion on waking and may be a sign of a separate form of idiopathic hypersomnia.

Heart rates of idiopathic hypersomniacs are higher than those of normal persons before and during sleep. Sleep recordings show that the sleep itself seems more aroused. The pattern of progression through 90-minute sleep cycles is normal, however, even in sleeps lasting 20 hours.

Methylphenidate or dextroamphetamine are prescribed for idiopathic hypersomniacs throughout the day. When taken at bedtime as well, these stimulants abolish sleep drunkenness on waking. To prevent sleep drunkenness and produce normal waking, another clinician has suggested rousing the sleeper sufficiently to take a dose of stimulant one hour before his normal waking time.

8. Abnormal Sleep-Wake Rhythms

Excessive daytime sleepiness may appear in persons whose natural, biological sleep-wake rhythms are chronically shifted out of phase with their social environments, or whose rhythms have cycles longer than the 24-hour cycles of normal persons. Patients are sometimes seen whose sleep-wake cycles are 25-27 hours in length, though cases with 36-38-hour cycles have been reported. These patients sleep normally, but do so at the "wrong" time relative to their social requirements. They are unable to maintain a "normal" 24-hour sleep-wake "day." Sleep clinicians are divided as to what treatment can be offered these persons. Research is under way at some sleep research centers to characterize these patients' problems.

Centers for the TM Program

The following are some of the major centers offering courses in the Transcendental Meditation Program.

UNITED STATES

Ann Arbor
1207 Packard
Ann Arbor, Mich. 48104
Phone: (313) 761-8255

Atlanta
3615 N. Stratford Road N.E.
Atlanta, Ga. 30342
Phone: (404) 231-1093

Baltimore
809 St. Paul Street
Baltimore, Md. 21202
Phone: (301) 837-6114

Berkeley
2716 Derby Street
Berkeley, Calif. 94705
Phone: (415) 548-1144

Boston
73 Newbury Street
Boston, Mass. 02116
Phone: (617) 266-3770

Cambridge
33 Garden Street
Cambridge, Mass. 02138
Phone: (617) 876-4581

Charlotte
1532 E. Morehead Street
Charlotte, N.C. 28207
Phone: (704) 332-6694

Chicago
145 E. Ohio
Chicago, Ill. 60611
Phone: (312) 467-5570

Cincinnati
3047 Madison Road
Cincinnati, Ohio 45209
Phone: (513) 631-6800

Columbus
1818 West Lane Ave.
Upper Arlington, Ohio 43221
Phone: (614) 481-8877

Dallas
3603 North Hall, Suite 204
Dallas, Tex. 75219
Phone: (214) 528-3600

Denver
215 St. Paul
#280
Denver, Colo. 80206
Phone: (303) 320-4007

Des Moines
1311 34th Street
Des Moines, Iowa 50311
Phone: (515) 255-2547

Detroit
17108 Mack at Cadieux
Grosse Pointe, Mich. 48230
Phone: (313) 885-5566

Greensboro
312 S. Aycock St.
Greensboro, N.C. 27403
Phone: (919) 275-2772

Hartford
299 Farmington Ave.
Hartford, Conn. 06105
Phone: (203) 246-8821

Honolulu
227 S. King Street
Honolulu, Hawaii 96813
Phone: (808) 537-3339

Houston
2518 Drexel
Houston, Tex. 77027
Phone: (713) 627-7500

Kansas City
6301 Main Street
Kansas City, Mo. 64113
Phone: (816) 523-5777

Los Angeles
1015 Gayley Avenue
Los Angeles, Calif. 90024
Phone: (213) 478-1569

Memphis
1639 Madison Avenue
Memphis, Tenn. 38104
Phone: (901) 726-6691

Miami
3251 Ponce de Leon Boulevard
Suite 210
Coral Gables, Fla. 33134
Phone: (305) 444-6172

Milwaukee
400 E. Silver Spring
Whitefish Bay, Wis. 53217
Phone: (414) 962-7560

Minneapolis
6524 Walker Street
Suite 212
Saint Louis Par, Minn. 55426
Phone: (612) 929-0071

New Haven
1974 Yale Station
New Haven, Conn. 06520
Phone: (203) 776-5784

New Orleans
2324 Napoleon Avenue
New Orleans, La. 70115
Phone: (504) 899-6380

New York
133 E. 58th Street
New York, N.Y. 10022
Phone: (212) 826-6620

Omaha
4202 Dodge Street
Suite 200
Omaha, Neb. 68131
Phone: (402) 551-1010

Philadelphia
315 S. 17th Street
Philadelphia, Pa. 19103
Phone: (215) 732-9220

Phoenix
2234 N. Seventh Street
Suite 2
Phoenix, Ariz. 85006
Phone: (602) 257-8611

Pittsburgh
5883 Forbes Avenue
Pittsburgh, Pa. 15217
Phone: (412) 521-6000

Portland
7743 S.W. Capitol Highway
Portland, Oregon 97219
Phone: (503) 245-3361

Richmond
1810 Monument Avenue
Richmond, Va. 23220
Phone: (804) 359-2772

Sacramento
2454 Loma Vista Dr.
Sacramento, Calif. 95825
Phone: (916) 485-5706

St. Louis
742 Emerson Road
St. Louis, Mo. 63141
Phone: (314) 569-0020

San Diego
2180 Garnet Ave.
#3-J
San Diego, Calif. 92109
Phone: (714) 270-7670

San Francisco
256 Laguna Honda Boulevard
San Francisco, Calif. 94116
Phone: (415) 661-7050

Seattle
912 15th Avenue E.
Seattle, Wash. 98105
Phone: (206) 322-1800

Tampa
10921 N. 56th Street
Suite 203
Temple Terrace, Fla. 33617
Phone: (813) 985-6733

Washington, D.C.
2127 Leroy Place, N.W.
Washington, D.C. 20008
Phone: (202) 387-5050

CANADA

Calgary
218-11th Avenue, S.W.
Calgary
Alberta T2R 0C3
Phone: (403) 262-1030

Edmonton
Le Marchand Mansions
101-11523 100th Avenue
Edmonton
Alberta T5K 0J8
Phone: (403) 482-1371

Halifax
2045 Poplar Street
Halifax
N.S. B3L 2Y6
Phone: (902) 422-5905

Hamilton
1960 Main Street W.
Hamilton
Ontario L9G 2V9
Phone: (416) 527-0444

Moncton
256 Cameron Street
Moncton
N.B. E1C 5Z3
Phone: (506) 855-0225

Montreal West
3666 Lorne Crescent
Montreal
P.Q. H2X 2B3
Phone: (514) 285-1298

Ottawa
65 Bank Street
Ottawa
Ontario K1P 5N2
Phone: (616) 236-0648

Quebec
1085 Avenue des Erables
Quebec
P.Q. G1R 2N3
Phone: (418) 529-2149

Regina
2326 Albert Street
Regina
Saskatchewan S4P 2V7
Phone: (306) 586-4012

Saskatoon
707 University Drive
Saskatoon
Saskatchewan S7W 0J3
Phone: (306) 242-6317

Sources for Herbs

Arizona

Idell Sales Co.
P.O. Box 634
Sedona, Arizona 86336

California

Lhasa Karnak Herb Co.
2482 Telegraph Avenue
Berkeley, California 94704

King's Herbs
471 E. Belmont Avenue
Fresno, California 93701

Basic Herb Headquarters
8501 S. Vermont
Los Angeles, California 90044

China Herb Company
428 Soledad
Salinas, California 93901

Nature's Herb Company
281 Ellis Street
San Francisco, California 94102

Colorado

American Tea, Coffee and Spice Co.
1511 Champa
Denver, Colorado 80202

Connecticut

Capriland's Herb Farm
Silver Street
Coventry, Connecticut 06238

Hart Seed Co. (herb seeds)
Main and Hart Streets
Wethersfield, Connecticut 06109

District of Columbia

The Herb Cottage
Washington Cathedral
Mount St. Alban
Washington, D.C. 20016

Illinois

National Herb Co.
512 N. LaSalle
Chicago, Illinois 60610

Indiana

Henderson's Botanical Gardens
Route 6
Greensburg, Indiana 47240

Maine

Merry Gardens
P.O. Box 595
Camden, Maine 04843

Maryland

Hahn and Hahn Homeopathic Pharmacy
324 W. Saratoga Street
Baltimore, Maryland 21201

Massachusetts

Cape Cod Nurseries (native live herbs)
P.O. Drawer B
Falmouth, Massachusetts 02541

The Herbery
Homestead Road, Box 543
Orleans, Massachusetts 02653

Michigan

Harvest Health, Inc.
1944 Eastern Avenue, S.E.
Grand Rapids, Michigan 49507

Minnesota

Ferndale Nursery and Greenhouse
P.O. Box 218
Askov, Minnesota 55704

Missouri

Wise's K.C. Homeopathic Pharmacy
4200 Lacleade Avenue
St. Louis, Missouri 63108

New Hampshire

Exeter Wildflower Gardens
P.O. Box 510
Exeter, New Hampshire 03883

New Jersey

House of Herbs
459 18th Avenue
Newark, New Jersey 07108

New York

Aphrodisia
28 Carmine Street
New York, New York 10014

Ye Olde Herbal Shoppe
8 Beekman
New York, New York 10038

Ohio

Hindue East Herb Co.
635 W. Court
Cincinnati, Ohio 45203

Oregon

Siskiyou Rare Plant Nursery (Herbs)
522 Franquette Street
Medford, Oregon 97501

Pennsylvania

The Rosemary House
Mechanicsburg, Pennsylvania 17055

Rhode Island

Greene Herb Gardens
Greene, Rhode Island 02898

Texas

Hilltop Herb Farm
P.O. Box 866
Cleveland, Texas 77327

Utah

Native Health Products
7200 South 2700 West
West Jordan, Utah 84084

Vermont

Bushacres Herb Farm
Brandon, Vermont 05733

Virginia

The Heritage Store
P.O. Box 444-A
Virginia Beach, Virginia 23458

Washington

The Wild Garden
P.O. Box 487
Bothell, Washington 98011

INDEX